A Psychologist's Proactive Guide to Managed Mental Health Care

A Psychologist's Proactive Guide to Managed Mental Health Care

Edited by

Alan J. Kent
PacMed Clinics, Seattle

Michel Hersen
Pacific University

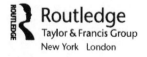

Routledge
Taylor & Francis Group
New York   London

First published by Lawrence Erlbaum Associates, Inc., Publishers
10 Industrial Avenue
Mahwah, New Jersey 07430

Reprinted 2009 by Routledge

Routledge

270 Madison Avenue
New York, NY 10016

2 Park Square, Milton Park
Abingdon, Oxon OX14 4RN, UK

Cover design by Kathryn Houghtaling Lacey

Library of Congress Cataloging-in-Publication Data

A psychologist's proactive guide to managed mental health care / edited
by Alan J. Kent, Michel Hersen.
    p. cm.
Includes bibliographical references and index.
    ISBN 0-8058-2910-5 (cloth : alk. paper) — ISBN 0-8058-3488-5 (pbk :
alk. paper)
    1. Clinical psychology—Practice—United States. 2. Managed mental
health care—United States. I. Kent, Alan J. II. Hersen, Michel.
RC467.95.P793 2000
362.2—dc21   99-16478
                                    CIP

10   9   8   7   6   5   4   3   2   1

Contents

Preface

The decade of the 1990s has witnessed a major revolution in health care that has had a staggering impact on all providers who have had to reconceptualize the vast majority of their assumptions about clinical care, how and when they deliver services, and how they are compensated for their activities. The impact has been profound and dramatic for providers in the mental health field in particular. In this book we focus on clinical and counseling psychologists.

Although many psychologists attribute the growing hegemony of managed care solely to the commercialization of the field, in reality several other factors have had an influence. Among them are the increased need for accountability in clinical practice, the exponential cost of providing health services, including mental health services, and the initial reluctance (and in some quarters continued resistance) of psychologists to constitute themselves part of the solution. That is, many psychologists and their professional organizations have struggled against the health maintenance organizations (HMOs) rather than working from within to influence their decision-making processes.

Hardly a week goes by now without some article by and for psychologists bemoaning their fates at the hands of managed care. However, this pessimistic attitude is exaggerated and in the long run unhealthy for the field. Rather, what is needed is a balanced approach that not only will prevent panic but that will help psychologists *capitalize on the new opportunities*. Our vision of a balanced approach guided our development of this book. To the reader, let us underscore that it is the *proactive* guide to managed mental health care.

The book is divided into three parts: Part I: General Issues of Managed Care, Part II: Modification of Traditional Roles Under Managed Care, and Part III: New Roles for Psychologists Under Managed Care.

In each of the chapters an optimistic and proactive approach to dealing with managed care and the new health care system is detailed. As the American icon Ann Landers has been quoted as saying, "When life deals you lemons, make lemonade." Therefore, in each of the chapters a noted expert has reviewed varied aspects of psychological practice and has given the reader a chance to see opportunities for professional growth and development. In Part I, in the first chapter, the editors present the overview of managed mental health care.

In Part II (chaps. 2–4) the authors focus on the traditional roles of psychologists in the United States and address the ways in which these roles have evolved in the era of managed mental health care. In chapter 2, William I. Dorfman, a professor of psychology, a published researcher on assessment, and a private practitioner, describes a new development in the arena of psychological assessment. Traditional assessment methods are being curtailed. However, there are many new possibilities for psychologists willing to alter their assessment practices. In chapter 3 Carol S. Austad describes changes in the practice of psychotherapy in the age of managed care. As an academician and a practitioner in one of the country's most well-known staff model HMOs, Dr. Austad is in a unique position to discuss new challenges and opportunities. In chapter 4, K. Roy MacKenzie describes the exciting changes and challenges facing group therapy practitioners in the current marketplace. He has written extensively on group therapy and has been actively researching and reviewing new models of treatment that are applicable to managed care.

Part III (chaps. 5–7) explores new and innovative roles for psychologists that have evolved in the new health care system and considers how psychologists can respond to the demands that are being placed on them. In chapter 5, Kurt Strosahl describes a creative and exciting new role for psychologists as behavioral health consultants in the primary health care delivery system. Kurt Strosahl is a manager in one of the nation's oldest and largest staff model HMOs and has written extensively about practice in the managed care era. In chapter 6, Hanna Levenson and Joanna Burg review some of their own research on training and point out clear directions for where the field needs to go if we are to train psychologists for the new millennium. Finally, in chapter 7, Nicholas A. Cummings, one of the true visionaries of American psychology, a former president of the American Psychological Association, a founder of the California School of Professional Psychology, and a founder of American Biodyne (one of the early mental health MCO giants), tells us where we have been, where we are going, and how psychology can keep up. The chapter reflects this author's cutting edge view of the mental health field.

Many people have contributed to the fruition of this book. First and foremost, we thank the eminent authors for taking time out from their busy schedules to share their thinking and expertise with us. Second, we thank Carole Londerée, Eleanor Gil, and Erika Qualls for their invaluable technical expertise. Finally, but hardly least of all, we thank Larry and our other friends at Lawrence Erlbaum Associates, Inc., for their willingness to undertake this timely project.

—Alan J. Kent, PhD, ABPP
Seattle, Washington
—Michel Hersen, PhD, ABPP
Forest Grove, Oregon

Part I

General Issues of Managed Care

An Overview of Managed Mental Health Care: Past, Present, and Future

Alan J. Kent
PacMed Clinics

Michel Hersen
Pacific University

By now it should be no surprise to any practicing psychologist that the mental health care field has changed enormously since the 1980s. Of course, these changes affecting professional psychology are just a part of the overall revamping of the American health care system. In the late 1980s, Zimet (1989) warned psychology of the coming changes in health care and urged psychologists to alter their perspective. He wrote, "The sooner we psychologists put aside our thinking that magically the situation will reverse itself and return to the free choice system that has been the standard for many years, the sooner we can deal in an adaptive manner with the radical changes that are occurring" (p. 705). He also urged psychologists to "take some control of managed health programs" (p. 707). At that time, he also lamented the fact that organized professional psychology had taken a position in opposition to managed care rather than try to make a place for psychologists in the managed care market.

Clearly, Zimet's forecast was correct. Although the American Psychological Association (APA) and other organizations predicted the demise of managed care, the number of Americans covered by managed mental health care organizations skyrocketed, so that as of 1998, more than 170 million lives are covered by these programs (Practice Strategies, 1998).

So much has been written about managed care since the late 1980s that literature searches on the topic now reveal hundreds of articles. There is much still much controversy about the utility and benefit of managed care systems, but few still argue that these systems will go away. There is no question that professional psychology has been profoundly affected by the changes in the health

3

care system. A review of guild publications reveals numerous "horror stories" about the decline of psychology. Mesh (1998) complained that recent psychology graduates are "all dressed up with nowhere to go" (p. 17). He described the plight of new psychology graduates who, if they are fortunate enough to find work, earn less than word processors. Other reports describe the plight of health maintenance organization (HMO) psychologists who are unionizing and staging strikes to protest low wages and poor working conditions (McGuire, 1998). As master's level therapists continue to grow in number and gain licensure and credibility with insurers and managed care companies, psychology must vie for position in the coming era. As Russ Newman, executive director for professional practice at the APA, has said, "If psychologists focus only on mental health assessment and psychotherapy, then, yes, there will be too many psychologists." (cited in Clay, 1998a, p. 20).

Opportunities do exist for psychology in the new health care system. However, we must take a proactive stance, examine our strengths and capabilities, and look toward the future rather than lament the past. As APA's Newman has said, "Psychologists should become well versed in the business of health care and look at ways they can diversify their practices" (cited in Martin, 1998, p. 44). Our book, therefore, is designed to help psychologists gain the insights and develop the tools needed to move forward in the new millennium.

HOW DID WE GET HERE?

In order to understand the current state of affairs in the U.S. health care system, it is important to have some background and understanding of how we arrived at this place. Although this has been reviewed extensively elsewhere (for instance, Austad & Berman, 1991; DeLeon, Bulatao, & VandenBos, 1991), it is necessary to provide a brief overview of the past.

Broskowkski (1991) provides an excellent early perspective on why managed care developed so quickly in this country. By the 1980s, health care costs had skyrocketed. Although they represented only 6% of the gross national product (GNP) in 1965, by the early 1990s they were approaching 15% of the GNP. Additionally, rate of spending on health care was nearly double the annual inflation rate. These costs did not go unnoticed by the government and private industry, the two primary payers for health care. As a result, several strategies were developed to contain health care costs, many of which were subsumed under the general heading of *managed care.*

Initially, mental health care was not fully included in the move toward managed care. However, as medical costs began to be reigned in, the increase in mental health care costs became more evident. One of the primary factors driving the increasing cost of in mental health services was the explosion in the number of for-profit private psychiatric beds in the country. As Broskowski (1991) reported, the number of private psychiatric hospitals grew from 180 to 250 in just 15 years. Psychologists who were practicing in the 1970s and 1980s likely remember the numerous inpatient adolescent treatment facilities that advertised for patients and typically had lengths of stay lasting 90 to 120 days. However, although inpatient costs made up the majority of the mental health care costs, insurers and employers were also skeptical of the ever increasing number of patients being seen for psychotherapy. One survey found that businesses spent $22 billion providing psychotherapy to employees in 1993, up 57% in just 5 years (Freudenheim, 1994). Employers had long been wary of psychotherapy, which seemed to have fuzzy outcomes and questionable benefit. As a result, mental health care began to receive the same scrutiny as other health services and the managed mental health care industry was born.

THE ALPHABET SOUP OF MANAGED CARE:
UNDERSTANDING THE BASICS

The term "managed care" is a complex one that actually incorporates many different types of delivery systems. Although many associate managed care with HMOs, this represents only one way of providing care. In addition to the HMO, which is the most common form of managed care, there is the Preferred Provider Organization (PPO) and the Independent Practice Association (IPA). Although a full review and description of these models is beyond the scope of this chapter, a brief summary is provided for the uninitiated reader.

HMOs were designed to offer patients affordable, prepaid, comprehensive health care. All care was managed by a primary care provider (PCP), which served as the gatekeeper of care. HMOs carefully monitored utilization and attempted to reduce the expenses of specialty care and hospitalizations. HMO utilization managers focused on limiting care to medically necessary treatments only. (A discussion of medical necessity as it relates to mental health follows.)

HMOs attempted to control financial incentives for overutilization by offering capitated payments to providers and fixed payments to hospitals. Capitation is a form of payment in which the provider receives a negotiated flat fee in exchange for providing all the patient's health care for the year. Capitation fees are often referred to by the acronym PMPM, which is the amount of money the provider receives per member per month. A provider that accepts capitation at risk agrees to provide all the necessary health care a patient needs during the course of the year and accepts the risk of losing money should the patient need excessive care. Obviously, under this system, the provider has a financial incentive for carefully monitoring care and reducing unnecessary utilization. Other forms of capitation may involve varying degrees of risk based on the nature of the contract the provider signs with the insurer.

Under capitation arrangements, HMOs developed elaborate systems for monitoring utilization. Utilization management (UM) often includes pretreatment authorization for access to specialty services and hospitalization and concurrent utilization for ongoing review of treatment plans. Most HMOs hire case or care managers to conduct utilization review. In the case of mental health services, UM is typically conducted by psychiatric nurses or social workers.

In the early days of managed care, HMOs were often developed as staff models, meaning that providers worked in clinics owned and managed by the insurance company. Over time, more managed care companies have moved to a network model, in which the insurer contracts with a network of community providers. In some cases, these network providers accept capitation payments and the associated risks. In other cases, providers are paid for their services at a discounted fee-for-service rate and agree to accept the stringent utilization management required by the company.

In reality, HMOs have been operating in this country providing care for special populations since the early 1900s (Austad & Berman, 1991). However, not until Congress passed the HMO Act of 1973 did the United States see significant development of these types of organizations. Such legislation and a series of subsequent measures were enacted in reaction to increasing health care costs and provided the funding and the impetus for the development of HMOs and the managed care industry.

PPOs represent an alternative way to manage care. They offer patients more flexibility in selecting providers but typically include many of the utilization management methods noted above. Providers that agree to participate in such networks typically are reimbursed at reduced fees and they also accept outside review of their work. Patients in PPOs may or may not be subject to the PCP gatekeeper, depending on the insurance contract.

Another system of care that has developed under managed care is the IPA. An IPA is a group of providers that form their own network of care, which can then contract with insurers for providing capitated care. IPAs are complex entities that can function in many different ways dependent on the nature of their incorporation. Typically, providers in IPAs operate out of their own offices and may provide care either on a discount fee-for-service basis or through a capitated risk contract.

THE RISE OF MANAGED MENTAL HEALTH CARE

In its infancy, many managed care programs integrated mental health care into the health care delivery system. Most early staff model HMOs offered mental health services in their clinics. Mental health providers were hired by the HMOs and these practitioners attempted to provide time-limited therapy to large populations of patients.

At the same time that HMOs developed staff clinics, some insurers developed PPO networks of mental health providers. There was little utilization management in the earlier days of PPO networks, but providers did agree to accept reduced reimbursement in exchange for being listed on the insurers network panel.

By the mid-1980s, many insurers had become frustrated with the increasing cost of mental health care and had difficulty managing these services. As a result, a new, more sophisticated industry of "carve-out" managed mental health care companies developed. These companies functioned as specialty providers to which the HMO insurer could literally carve out the mental health benefit. These independent managed care organizations (MCOs), which specialized in mental health and chemical dependency services, grew rapidly in the early 1990s. Many of these companies became successful and profitable, and eventually were purchased by larger companies or merged with existing insurers. At times, the growth of these MCOs was dizzying to practitioners trying to keep up with changes in the industry.

The managed mental health care industry developed a system of care that was parallel to the health care alternatives established by the large insurers. Many of the early industry giants (including American Biodyne, American Psych Management, U.S. Behavioral Health, and Human Affairs International) established their own mental health networks and some established staff model clinics. The large insurance companies became increasingly satisfied to carve out their mental health care to these specialty companies, and the industry grew rapidly. Before long, mental health providers experienced the same upheaval that their medical counterparts had been dealing with for some time.

THE IMPACT OF MANAGED MENTAL HEALTH CARE ON PSYCHOLOGY

It is no surprise that managed care has tremendously impacted the delivery of psychological services in this country. An objective review of the past 10 years of managed care reveals some positive and negative effects.

THE CHALLENGES

Any private practitioner of psychology can readily identify a litany of complaints about managed care and the impact it has had on the profession. The clearest concern has been managed care's intrusion into the therapy process. No longer can the psychologist develop a treatment plan with a patient and carry it out in without intrusion (if one expects a third party to pay for it). The reality is that the therapy relationship is no longer quite as sacrosanct as it had been. Third-party reviewers ask questions and demand answers when they are asked to foot the bill. Psychologists have clearly lost a degree of autonomy in their style of practice.

What makes matters more difficult for many psychologists is that their training and clinical orientation are contradictory to the managed care philosophy. Many psychologists are unable and unwilling to develop objective, behaviorally focused treatment plans or establish clear, measurable goals. For many psychodynamic practitioners, the basic principles that guide the managed care clinical model are seriously flawed. For a discussion of this issue, see Karon (1995) and Miller (1996).

Clinical Challenges

The clearest challenge that psychologists have faced as a result of managed care is the change in the way they have practiced the basic tools of the trade: assessment and psychotherapy. Not only have psychologists lost autonomy, but many have had to learn new ways to practice. (For an excellent discussion of these issues, see Austad, 1992; Hoyt, 1992).

In terms of assessment, most psychologists were accustomed to being able to conduct any kind of clinical assessment they felt was appropriate. If a therapist needed additional clinical information, psychological testing was performed. Full test batteries were often utilized, especially with children and adolescents. In the era of managed care, psychologists cannot expect that psychological testing will be routinely authorized. MCOs require significant justification and documentation to warrant psychological testing. In many cases, less expensive alternatives are sought. MCOs often apply the standards of a cost–benefit analysis to determine whether the value added by testing warrants the increase in costs. This can certainly be frustrating to the psychologist who has been accustomed to performing assessments at will.

The most significant impact on psychological practice as a result of managed care has been the change in the way therapy is authorized and provided under managed care. The key factor in all managed mental health care programs is the emphasis on brief treatment models. A minority of practicing psychologists in this country were specifically trained in models of time-limited therapy. In fact, many surveys suggest that training in brief therapy is sorely lacking, even today (Kent, 1995).

Much research suggests that the majority of therapy provided in this country is short term. Although this has been defined in many ways, surveys typically reveal that the average number of treatment visits is less than 12 (Budman & Gurman, 1988). However, many practicing psychologists were trained in long term therapy models or time-unlimited models. As a result, they have had great difficulty adjusting to the demands imposed by managed care.

There is an extensive body of literature that examines the variety of brief treatment models (see Budman, 1981; Wells & Gianetti, 1990). There are even newer models proposed that explicitly address the demands of conducting psychotherapy within an HMO. Austad & Berman (1991) coined the term "HMO therapy" to describe a set of skills and techniques that can be particularly useful in the HMO setting.

Despite the ample literature available and the plethora of continuing education workshops on the market, many psychologists have had difficulty developing the skills necessary to provide treatment in the era of managed care. Budman and Armstrong (1992), Nahmias (1992), and others have addressed the training needs of psychologists, but some have simply not been willing or able to accomplish such retraining.

In addition to the challenge brought on by the emphasis on time-limited therapy, many psychologists have been poorly prepared for dealing with the emphasis of MCOs on group treatment. In the high-volume world of HMOs and the pressures of finances brought about by capitated contracts, therapists are seeing a resurgence of interest in group therapy. Simply stated, group psychotherapy offers a clinically proven and cost-effective way to provide treatment to large populations. In many staff model HMOs, groups have been the treatment of choice. Group therapy allows HMOs with high demand to reach patients quicker and improve access without increasing staffing costs. Many patients respond well to groups and there is certainly much literature to support the effectiveness of this modality.

Unfortunately, many psychologists are unfamiliar with group treatment and unprepared for conducting significant numbers of groups. Certainly, the majority of private psychology practices do not routinely offer groups. Many barriers to the establishment of such groups exist (MacKenzie, 1994); these will be discussed in depth in chapter 4. However, at this point, it is significant to note that increased pressure to provide group treatment has produced difficulties for some psychologists. Most training programs in psychology give little attention to group modalities and often see it as an adjunct to individual treatment. In the era of managed care, group therapy is increasingly becoming the treatment of choice, and psychologists need to develop group skills in order to participate.

Administrative Challenges

In addition to the clinical concerns just noted, psychologists face significant administrative burdens under managed care. Most notable is the challenge that utilization review presents to the practitioner. Clinical care reviews by the MCOs can be time consuming and tedious. Providers must often become acquainted with a variety of care review procedures, forms, and guidelines. Even the solo practitioner now must rely on fax machines, computers, billing systems, and telephone pagers. Many practices cannot survive the new marketplace without full-time secretarial support. All these requirements add significant amounts to the overhead for maintaining a practice.

At the same time that expenses and costs are increasing, reimbursements for psychological services are declining. A recent survey by Saeman (1998) indicated that psychologists' incomes have plummeted in recent years. MCOs are under increasing pressure from employers and other payers to reduce premiums and costs, and, as a result, there is continuing downward pressure on fees. Additionally, with frequent mergers in the managed care industry (see Cummings, 1995, chap. 7) there are fewer and larger players who then have the ability to drive reimbursements even lower. It does not seem likely that this trend will change in the near future.

The growth of managed care has produced challenges for psychologists who have had very limited business or administrative skills. Many solo practitioners or small group practices survived for years without any administrative support. Patients often paid for psychological services up front and then submitted their own bills to seek insurance company reimbursement. Psychologists were able to focus exclusively on their clinical work, with few administrative headaches.

It is the rare practitioner who has been adequately prepared for dealing with network managers, capitation contracts, IPAs, case rates, and the like. Few, if any, graduate training programs address issues of practice management or teach the business skills needed in the current marketplace. As Levinson discusses in her chapter, even today, training in business and administrative skills is lacking in the current curriculum of most graduate psychology programs. Even new graduates of Psy.D. programs are poorly prepared to face current practice challenges.

Professional Challenges

While the pressure on the practitioner has grown, so too has the impact on the field as a whole. Although there is some debate about whether there is surplus of psychologists in the United States, it is evident that the number of doctoral and master's level providers has grown enormously since the early 1990s (Clay, 1998b). Doctoral level psychologists have never successfully demonstrated that they produce better therapy outcomes than master's providers. Therefore, as the supply of practitioners increases, MCOs tend to utilize lower paid master's level providers. In some markets, psychologists are increasingly being shut out of the managed care referral networks.

THE OPPORTUNITIES

Although it is clear that the new era in health care has had a powerful impact on professional psychology, not all of it has been negative. In what follows we identify some of the positive aspects of managed care.

Managed care has forced mental health practitioners to examine the way they practice their profession. Although we expect that most psychologists act for the good of their patients, it is clear that the old fee-for-service system had incentives that were geared toward the provision of unnecessary services. The new system of care demands that providers be accountable for their treatment.

In the 1970s and early 1980s, in the heyday of mental health reimbursements, there were notable abuses in the system. It was not unusual for patients to be needlessly admitted to psychiatric facilities for disorders that could easily be managed on an outpatient basis. It was also not uncommon to find patients engaged in interminable psychotherapy with little or no progress being made. Additionally, overutilization of psychological testing by unscrupulous practitioners was evident (Kent, 1993).

Managed care utilization monitors have forced professionals to be accountable for their treatment decisions. Care managers scrutinize treatment plans and ask questions that require providers to think about their assumptions and approaches to treatment. There is increasing support and encouragement for the use of empirically validated treatments that give patients access to research-based interventions (Giles, 1991). Through care management, there is also greater opportunity to integrate mental health care with physical care. Furthermore, it is more difficult for substance-abusing patients to access multiple providers for medications or to avoid treatment. Managed care has the potential to provide better integration in mental health services.

Another benefit to grow out of managed care is the emergence of new schools of time-limited and briefer psychotherapies (Hoyt, 1992). As managed care companies have focused on more cost containment, they have demanded more effective and efficient models of care. Although briefer treatment models predate the managed care industry (see Budman & Gurman, 1988), not until the advent of carve-out MCOs did we see such an explosion in research and writing on brief treatment. Mental health practitioners had been complacent in the prevailing psychodynamic perspective, which believes that long-term therapy is the only adequate approach. The public has benefited by this access to brief therapy, which is clearly supported by the literature (Budman & Gurman, 1988).

Managed care has also benefited consumers in other ways. In the past, only those with significant resources could access psychotherapy. With the advent of the HMO, many more people now have access to psychological services. Although the benefit may be limited and the care may be reviewed, a whole new population can now have the opportunity to see a psychologist when needed. At the same time, psychologists have access to a large new patient base. Those psychologists who have the necessary skills to work comfortably with managed care companies can see their referrals grow (Sabin, 1991).

The growth and development of the managed care industry has given psychologists new opportunities for employment and professional growth (Cummings, 1995; Hersch, 1995). Many MCOs look to psychologists for the breadth of their training and experience. Psychologists function as clinical managers, supervisors, and directors in many different settings in the health care system. For those psychologists who seek applied work and do not want to do psychotherapy on a full-time basis, managed care companies offer a range of professional options. Additionally, for those who obtain the needed business skills, ample opportunities exist for well-trained psychologists as middle managers and directors in the managed care field. Many psychologists have sought additional training in health care management, and some have obtained master of business administration degrees to become high-level managers in the industry.

Although managed care companies have been utilizing the skills of master's level providers with more regularity, psychologists are more likely to be used as clinical supervisors and clinical planners. Psychologists have been carving out a niche in MCOs by developing treatment guidelines, supervising masters clinicians, reviewing clinical programs, and providing training and education to lower level providers and MCO staff.

In the past, psychological research in mental health was typically limited to academia and Veterans Administration medical centers. With the advent of the managed mental health company, psychologists are being called on to develop applied research programs, examining topics as diverse as consumer satisfaction and patient outcomes. As managed care companies are subjected to increasing requirements from accrediting bodies, it is expected that psychologists will be called on to help develop evaluation programs and data collection systems (Belar, 1989).

THE NEXT GENERATION OF MANAGED CARE

In the early days of managed care, profits were high for those MCOs and start-up mental health companies that made drastic cuts in the cost of mental health care. Employers and payers were delighted when mental health costs declined dramatically. Recent evidence reveals that development of managed care systems had a far greater impact on reducing the cost of mental health care than it did on health care in general. One recent report by the Hay Group consulting firm suggested that mental health care costs were cut by 54% in the same time that medical costs declined by only 7% (Hendren, 1998). However, by 1998, most of the "fat" had been removed from the mental health care system. Inpatient psychiatric hospitalizations have decreased, numerous private psychiatric and chemical dependency programs have closed, the majority of Americans receive their mental health care in managed programs, and reimbursement rates for providers remain at levels from the 1980s.

As MCOs merge and profit margins decline, there is little room to squeeze more savings from the system. At the same time, consumer backlash is evident with increasing calls for new legislation designed to reign in the excesses of managed care. As of this writing, there is strong indication that we will see a so-called "patients' bill of rights" in the near future.

In addition, recent years have also witnessed the passage of mental health parity laws throughout the country. On the surface, these well-intentioned laws are designed to eliminate discrimination against the mentally ill and ensure that those people with chronic psychiatric illnesses are able to obtain needed care. In fact, parity laws may actually increase involvement of managed care companies because employers fear costs of unlimited mental health benefit packages.

Because parity prohibits insurers from establishing separate dollar limits for medical and psychiatric illnesses, most companies have sidestepped the provision by redefining benefit packages. Now, instead of having $2,000 annual limit for outpatient mental health care, many plans insert annual session limits (e.g., 20 visits per year, up to $100 paid per visit).

FOCUS ON QUALITY

As a result of consumer advocacy and political pressures, the managed care industry is undergoing change. No longer is cost the only variable that drives employer contracts. Although purchasers of health care remain very sensitive to price, they are also demanding quality care and demonstrable outcomes.

The managed care industry is now faced with increasing pressure to spend more effort managing care rather than just cost. Most surviving managed care companies have expensive quality improvement departments, with elaborate data collection and information systems. Purchasers are also looking to accrediting bodies to evaluate and monitor health insurers and MCOs.

In the past, the Joint Commission on the Accreditation of Health Care Organizations represented the "gold standard" of accrediting bodies in health care. Today, the National Commission on Quality Assurance (NCQA) is the entity that has the most profound impact on MCOs. The NCQA is considered by many to be the essential seal of approval for any MCO. Until recently, NCQA focused on medical organizations, but it has recently released standards for accrediting managed mental health organizations.

Of course, increasing pressure on MCOs is transferred on to providers. Those psychologists who work extensively with managed care have become increasingly familiar with new standards regarding access to care, after-hours services, documentation, outcome, and peer review of care.

It is now commonplace for psychologists on managed care panels to be expected to have access standards that allow for patients to be seen for an initial visit within 48 hours. MCOs also require 24-hour phone coverage for emergencies and insist that patients in crisis be seen the same day. Practitioners also receive detailed guidelines about clinical documentation that specify what must be included in an initial evaluation and in a progress note. MCO reviewers often request complete copies of records to assess compliance with NCQA and company standards.

FOCUS ON OUTCOMES

Another major focus in this new era of managed care is the emphasis on outcomes. In the past, psychologists conducted their treatment and ideally terminated with the patient when there was mutual agreement on the progress made. Today, purchasers and insurers demand more concrete evidence of the effectiveness of treatment. Practitioners are expected to utilize standardized measures, surveys, or checklists to assess patient progress. MCOs then evaluate providers based on the success they achieve with patients.

Providers themselves are routinely evaluated by patients and MCOs. In the early days of the industry, the focus was on finding providers who kept treatment visits low and who infrequently hospitalized patients. Although these are still important considerations for network managers, companies are also asking patients to complete routine consumer satisfaction surveys that rate everything from the friendliness of support staff to the cleanliness of the office. As networks grow larger and the number of companies grows smaller, MCOs need to rely on aggregate patient satisfaction data to assess their network and comply with NCQA standards.

THE ADVENT OF PRACTICE GUIDELINES

One of the most dramatic trends in the industry relates to the development of practice guidelines. For decades, psychologists worked alone in their offices with their patients and little was actually known about what occurred behind the consultation room. Each psychologist had his or her manner and style of practice based on training, personality, and so on. These days, purchasers of health care want to see some standardization of practices, with an emphasis on empirically validated treatments. Third-party payers have long been skeptical of the vague nature of psychotherapy, especially the traditional psychodynamic approach. Now, largely as a result of an impressive body of psychological literature, information about what type of treatment works for what type of patient in what situation is available. There is no shortage of evidence as to the effectiveness of psychotherapy. Purchasers now insist that they will pay only for treatments that are known to be effective.

MCOs long ago stopped paying for nondirective or growth-oriented psychotherapy. Since the inception of managed care, the emphasis has been placed on reimbursing practitioners for *medically necessary* treatment. Although this term was often vague and unclear when applied to mental health, purchasers are now clear about this issue. Psychotherapy is reimbursed if it is utilized for treating a psychiatric illness as defined by the DSM-IV. Furthermore, in an increasing number of cases, MCOs are identifying the types of treatment that will be reimbursed and developing guidelines for how to apply these treatments to specific populations. These guidelines, which are often referred to as "practice guidelines" or "best practices," are increasingly becoming the industry standard.

Some managed care companies are developing their own guidelines with the assistance of their clinical staff or consultants. Other companies simply incorporate published treatment guidelines developed by organizations such as the American Academy of Child Psychiatry or the American Psychiatric Association. In either case, psychologists who practice in MCO networks are expected to adhere to the guidelines adapted by the company. Purchasers of care are not only managing the length of treatment and the level of care provided, but also specifying the type of care that they will reimburse.

In practice, this has had a great impact on both patients and providers. The senior author has worked with a patient who had a serious major depressive disorder but was unwilling to seek a psychiatric evaluation or take antidepressants. After several months of outpatient psychotherapy, the managed care company refused to reimburse additional psychotherapy visits unless the patient complied with its insistence on a psychiatric evaluation.

One may argue about whether this is appropriate or ethical on the part of the managed care company. However, at the bottom line, when the company is paying for the service, it does have some right to dictate the terms. At a clinical level, such intrusion in the consultation room may ultimately help patients by forcing providers to stay abreast of the literature and to utilize known effective techniques. Regardless of how one feels about such practice guidelines, they are clearly being implemented around the country and they represent an aspect of care that psychologists need to be prepared to address.

SHIFTING RISK

Since inception of managed care, most of the financial risk involved in providing care has been placed on the insurers and the managed mental health carveout companies. PCPs often shared the financial risk of providing medical care by accepting capitation rates. However, capitation has not generally trickled down to the mental health care provider.

Until more recently, psychologists faced the financial burden of reduced reimbursements that were reflective of the financial risks taken by the mental health MCOs. However, the larger MCOs have moved in the direction of sharing the risk with the providers themselves. Although this had been done with PCPs for some time, it is a newer concept for psychologists to deal with.

Many providers and patients have complained about the clinical micromanagement of cases that some MCOs engage in. Additionally, there is a significant cost associated with doing clinical reviews and utilization management. By sharing the financial risk with the provider, the MCO is able to reduce its administrative overhead and satisfy providers' demand for more autonomy.

Risk sharing in mental health typically takes two forms: capitation and case rates. As discussed earlier, capitation is a form of reimbursement in which the provider group is paid a flat fee, per member per month, to provide care for a given population. In some cases, the capitation is known as *full risk,* in which the mental health provider is responsible for managing all levels of care, including inpatient, outpatient, and pharmacology. In other cases, the provider group may be capitated only for the outpatient therapy. In either case, only well-organized service systems and provider groups are able to successfully manage capitated contracts. Typically, mental health MCOs have entered into capitated agreements with IPAs and integrated delivery systems (IDS; see below). Development of capitated contracts requires a good deal of business acumen and knowledge on behalf of the psychologist or provider group. To date, these type of capitation arrangements appear to be on the rise as more IPAs develop the capability to manage them.

A simpler form of risk sharing involves the application of case rates. Whereas capitation involves prepayment for an entire defined population, case rates represent prepayment for a specific patient or diagnostic group. In the case rate model of reimbursement, patients referred to a particular provider are paid a flat fee for the treatment of the patient. In some instances, the case rate reflects a time period (e.g., all outpatient treatment for the year); in other instances, it may apply to a specific episode of care (e.g., until the anxiety remits). As of this writing, we are aware that some MCOs are offering psychologists fees of $200 to $240 per year for the treatment of an outpatient, and some IPAs and community mental health centers are receiving a case rate of several thousand dollars per year to manage a patient with schizophrenia.

Although this form of reimbursement may seem unique and intimidating to the psychologist, it has been around for some time in the medical field. In the 1980s, the Medicare program began reimbursing hospitals based on diagnostic related groups. Under this form of payment, a hospital was paid a flat fee for a particular diagnosis, regardless of the actual length of stay. Until recently, this approach was not applied to mental health conditions. Introduction of case rates suggests that we will likely see more attempts to apply prepayment for psychiatric conditions.

In both the case rate and the capitation model, the provider becomes the manager of the clinical care. The provider has the financial risk as well as the incentive to treat the patients in the most cost-effective manner. In exchange for less outside intrusion from managed care reviewers, the provider now has intrinsic motivation to develop innovative treatment approaches to ensure that patients are cared for in a clinically appropriate and cost-effective manner. On a practice level, this translates into using more time-limited therapies, developing group interventions, seeking to avoid costly inpatient care, and providing access to crisis intervention.

Some psychologists may find this approach abhorrent and feel that they do not want to be faced with the ethical dilemmas inherent in such a system. From the MCO perspective, however, it makes sense to realign the financial incentives. Under the old health care model, providers had an incentive to provide as much care as possible, often overutilizing services. Now, providers are forced to apply their clinical principles to a system that has a direct financial impact on them.

Clearly, risk-sharing models are not for everyone and they are certainly difficult to manage in a solo practice or small office. As a result, new care delivery systems that enable providers to meet the demands of the new generation of managed care are being developed.

INTEGRATED DELIVERY SYSTEMS

Until the mid-1980s, most outpatient mental health care was provided by solo practitioners or in small offices. With the exception of federally funded community mental health centers and family counseling agencies, few psychologists practiced in group settings. With the advent of managed care and the burdens associated with it, mental health practice groups have grown exponentially in this country. Some observers have even predicted the demise of the solo practice (Cummings, Pallak, & Cummings, 1996).

Increasingly, mental health MCOs have moved in the direction of contracting with group practices rather than with solo practitioners. MCO network managers have learned that it is more effective to manage a network composed of a handful of large, well-organized groups rather than dozens of individual practitioners. Furthermore, group practices often have the administrative structure that allows them to perform needed quality improvement and data collection activities. As previously discussed, group practices are also more likely to have the capability to take on risk-sharing contracts.

Traditionally, mental health MCOs have maintained carve-out contracts with insurance companies. MCOs then, in turn, have contracted with networks of mental health providers. However, increasingly the trend is for mental health organizations to band together with medical providers and inpatient hospitals to form IDSs.

In an IDS, the provider group can offer a comprehensive range of medical and mental health services that can contract directly with insurance companies and/or purchasers (employers). Such arrangements can effectively eliminate the middle man, or the managed mental health company.

IDSs make sense when one examines the literature in medical cost offset. An ample body of research supports the fact that access to mental health services can reduce unnecessary utilization of medical services. Additionally, estimates suggest that anywhere from 30% to 60% of primary care visits are related to psychosocial issues. Finally, numerous surveys show that most psychotropic medication is prescribed by primary care doctors, not by psychiatrists (Selen, 1997). By developing IDSs, health care providers can more easily facilitate the total mind/body integration of health care.

Under the carve out model of mental health care, patients could potentially be bounced back and forth from medical to mental health systems, each with a different set of financial incentives. For instance, if the PCP is not capitated for mental health, why not immediately refer the depressed patient to the mental health provider? If the mental health MCO is carved-out, why not refer the patient back to the PCP for any physical complaints? This conflict is most evident in treatment of patients with those disorders that most clearly straddle the mind/body boundary such as eating disorders, organic brain disorders, and the like.

The trend toward integration of medical and mental health has a profound impact for psychologists (Hersch, 1995). As discussed by Strosahl in chapter 5, psychologists can play unique roles in this integrated system. Psychologists have the opportunity to work closely with medical providers, addressing issues in behavioral medicine, wellness, and prevention.

The trend toward IDS does have some mental health MCOs concerned. The industry has grown so rapidly and is founded on the carve-out concept. As integration becomes the buzzword, mental health MCOs will be looking for new ways to deliver care.

SUMMARY

The changes in the mental health care field over the past two decades are truly astounding. The health care system in the United States continues to evolve. None of the stakeholders in the system (consumers, providers, purchasers, payers) appears satisfied with the current situation, and it is difficult to predict what the future holds.

As psychologists, we have not been very successful in fighting the changes to date. It is unlikely that these changes will be reversed; there is virtually no chance that the profession will return to the days of unrestricted reimbursement and long-term therapy for all.

However, when one reviews the entire picture, it is evident that many of the changes have had a positive impact on our health care system and on our profession. Although psychologists face significant professional challenges, with these challenges come also exciting opportunities for growth and development if we are not afraid to face them (Broskowski, 1995).

REFERENCES

Austad, C. (1992). Managed health care and its effects on the practice of psychotherapy: Pros and cons. *Psychotherapy in Private Practice, 11*, 11–15.

Austad, C., & Berman, W. (1991). Managed care and the evolution of psychotherapy. In C. Austad. & W. Berman (Eds.), *Psychotherapy in managed health care: The optimal use of time and resources* (pp. 1–18). Washington, DC: American Psychological Association.

Belar, C. (1989). Opportunities for psychologists in health maintenance organizations: Implications for graduate education and training. *Professional Psychology: Research and Practice, 20,* 390–394.

Broskowski, A. (1991). Current mental health care environments: Why managed care is necessary. *Professional Psychology: Research and Practice, 22,*1–9.

Broskowski, A. (1995). The evolution of health care: Implications for training and careers of psychologists. *Professional Psychology: Research and Practice, 26,* 156–162.

Budman, S. (1981). *Forms of brief therapy.* New York: Guilford Press.

Budman, S., & Armstrong, E. (1992). Training for managed care settings: How to make it happen. *Psychotherapy, 29,* 416–421.

Budman, S., & Gurman, A. (1988). *The theory and practice of brief psychotherapy.* New York: Guilford Press.

Clay, R. (1998a, September). Mental health professions vie for position in the next decade. *APA Monitor,* 20–21.

Clay, R. (1998b, September). Psychologists, social workers and psychiatrists: Too many or not enough? *APA Monitor,* 20.

Cummings, N. (1995) Impact of managed care on employment and training: A primer for survival. *Professional Psychology: Research and Practice, 26,* 10–15.

Cummings, N., Pallak, M., & Cummings, J. (1996). *Surviving the demise of solo practice.* Madison, CT: Psychosocial Press.

DeLeon, P., Bulatao, E., & VandenBos, G. (1991). Managed mental health care: A history of the federal policy initiative. *Professional Psychology: Research and Practice, 22,* 15–25.

Freudenheim, M. (1994, April 12). Business using therapy data to lower costs. *New York Times,* p. C1.

Giles, T. (1991). Managed mental health care and effective psychotherapy: A step in the right direction? *Journal of Behavior Therapy and Experimental Psychiatry, 22,* 83–86.

Hendren, J. (1998, August 10). Bosses limit visits to therapists, skirt mental health law. *Seattle Times,* p. 8.

Hersch, L. (1995). Adapting to health care reform and managed care: Three strategies for survival and growth. *Professional Psychology: Research and Practice, 26,* 16–26.

Hoyt, M. (1992). Discussion of the effects of managed care on mental health practice. *Psychotherapy in Private Practice, 11,* 79–83.

Karon, B. (1995). Provision of psychotherapy under managed health care: A growing crisis and national nightmare. *Professional Psychology: Research and Practice, 26,* 5–9.

Kent, A. (1993). On psychology, ethics, and health care reform. *Psychotherapy Bulletin, 28*, 29–31.

Kent, A. (1995). *Training psychologists in brief therapy and managed care.* Paper presented at the 103rd Annual Convention of the American Psychological Association, New York.

MacKenzie, K. (1994). Where is here and when is now: The adaptational challenge of mental health reform for group psychotherapy. *International Journal for Group Psychotherapy, 44,* 407–427.

Martin, S. (1998, October). Willingness to diversify leads to practice success. *APA Monitor,* 44.

McGuire, P. (1998, September). Kaiser therapists stage one day strike. *APA Monitor,* 22.

Mesh, S. (1998, September). The plight of recent graduates: All dressed up with no where to go. *National Psychologist,* 17.

Miller, I. (1996). Some "short-term therapy values" are a formula for invisible rationing. *Professional Psychology: Research and Practice, 27,* 577–582.

Nahmias, V. (1992). Training for a managed care setting. *Psychotherapy in Private Practice, 11,* 15–19.

Is big better? (1998). *Practice Strategies, 4*(1), 1.

Sabin, J. (1991). Clinical skills for the 1990s: Six lessons from HMO practice. Hospital and *Community Psychiatry, 42,* 605–608.

Saeman, H. (1998, July/August). Survey: Psychologist's incomes plummet. *National Psychologist,* 1.

Selen, D. (1997). Integration of primary care and behavioral health: The driving forces. In J. Haber & G. Mitchell (Eds.), *Primary care meets mental health: Tools for the 21st century.* Tiburon, CA: Centralink Publications.

Wells, R. A., & Gianetti, V. J. (Eds.). (1990). *Handbook of the brief therapies.* New York: Plenum Press.

Zimet, C. (1989). The mental health care revolution: Will psychology survive. *American Psychologist, 44,* 703–708.

Part II

Modification of Traditional Roles Under Managed Care

Psychological Assessment and Testing Under Managed Care

William I. Dorfman
Nova Southeastern University

Since the mid-1980s, psychologists, as well as other mental health practitioners, have experienced a revolutionary shift in the way their profession is practiced, financially supported, and administratively controlled. Historically, psychologists have been accustomed to assuming full responsibility for all treatment decisions in terms of the type of therapy delivered, its length, and any assessment procedures utilized. Costs were passed on to traditional indemnity payers and practitioners often had little interest or incentive to control costs, limit services, or involve any third parties in the management of their patients. As health care costs have continued to spiral out of control, more than doubling the rate of inflation (Resnick & DeLeon, 1995), managed care organizations (MCOs) have dramatically expanded, covering increasing numbers of patient lives. Through a variety of organizational structures, MCOs have sought to address the financial health care crisis by administering mental health benefits in the most cost-effective manner possible, attempting to control costs while maintaining the quality and effectiveness of the services rendered. To these ends, many clinical decisions about patient care have shifted from the psychologist to the MCO case manager, often in partnership with company accounting executives. These decisions frequently have involved the elimination or attenuation of what administrators feel are ineffective or "medically unnecessary" services. Perhaps nowhere has the impact of these changes on psychologists been greater than on the practice of evaluation and testing.

Historically, psychological testing has been the "bread and butter" of clinical psychology and a key to its identity (American Psychological Association Clinical Division 12, 1993). Psychologists have been accustomed to viewing pretreatment evaluation and testing as integral parts of their case conceptualization and diagnosis, informing them about patients cognitive and personality

23

functioning, and directing the focus and course of treatment. In a managed care environment in which treatment sessions are often reduced, benefits are limited, and cost-benefit analysis is applied to all treatment authorizations, psychologists have been forced to justify the need and efficacy of their diagnostic procedures and to reevaluate the overall management of their patients.

Frequently, careful pretreatment evaluation, including testing, is eliminated when total sessions for the patient may number only four to eight visits. Case managers are responsible for extending benefits in the most efficient and effective manner and often are not persuaded that testing results in demonstrable gains for their clients. This problem is exacerbated by the fact that for the most part, case managers are not psychologists and have little experience with or knowledge about testing. Additionally, other mental health providers, including social workers, counselors, and psychiatrists, may provide many of the same treatment services without the benefit (or the unnecessary cost) of traditional psychological assessment. It is rare for psychologists to receive referrals from other professionals or from the MCO itself expressly to test patients prior to treatment. Although this situation is quite common in managed care, it is by no means universal. Each benefit plan and organizational structure—health maintenance organization, preferred provider organization, point of service, or exclusive provider organization, to name a few—has different sets of regulations and benefit packages. Psychologists must research each company separately and be knowledgeable about the benefit packages and limitations of each, particularly with reference to psychological testing. A review of the specific types of MCOs, their overall structures, and their philosophies of reimbursement is beyond the scope of this chapter.

SELLING TESTING TO MANAGED CARE

Within today's managed care environment, the psychologist's decision to utilize psychological assessment and evaluation in clinical practice is predicated on at least two practical considerations: (a) Will the use of evaluation and testing lead to demonstrable differences in the length and effectiveness of treatment? (b) Will the MCO pay for it? Obviously, for the practicing psychologist, these questions are interrelated and can be viewed within the framework of cost-benefit analysis. Can the benefits of psychological testing and evaluation be shown empirically to outweigh the costs of these procedures? Klump and Butcher (1997) point out that adequate research literature in support of such benefits has yet to materialize. The role of psychologists in empirically demonstrating positive treatment outcome, patient satisfaction, and other benefits of testing related to medical care is discussed later.

Until the value of testing can be shown unequivocally, support and reimbursement for evaluation and testing will be uneven within MCOs and frequently based on the psychologist's personal credibility and competence in justifying such expenditures. In the interim, it is incumbent on each psychologist to be aware of the goals and philosophy of the managed care industry, and to understand how the use of evaluation and testing with his or her patients not only is consistent with, but also helps to further, those goals. To the extent that these procedures can be shown to enhance the value of the managed care product by ensuring quality care and positive treatment outcome, to reduce treatment length without sacrificing that quality, to prevent overutilization of limited resources and services, and to enhance patient satisfaction with care, psychologists can expect to gain greater support for their unique testing skills from the managed care industry.

TRADITIONAL ROLES FOR PSYCHOLOGICAL TESTING

MCOs are sensitive to the needs of both the individual patient and the client organizations that typically purchase the insurance plans for their employees. Demands for specific services from these groups help to insure the inclusion of services (e.g., evaluation and testing) into the benefit package. Although testing benefits are clearly limited in most plans, MCOs are likely to include some traditional psychodiagnostic services in their plans in response to marketplace demands in order to ensure a competitive edge and maintain the value of their package. Neuropsychological evaluation, for instance, has become a highly specialized area, and qualified psychologists are likely to be successful in justifying this service to the case manager as medically necessary. Although extensive assessment with neuropsychological batteries, including the Halstead–Reitan (Reitan & Wolfson, 1993) or the Luria Nebraska (Golden, Hammeke, & Purisch, 1980), may be financially prohibitive, tailored screening batteries targeted to specific referral questions are more likely to be approved. Components of the Wechsler Adult Intelligence Scale-III (Psychological Corporation, 1998), Wechsler Memory Scale-III (Psychological Corporation), the Wisconsin Card Sort (Psychological Corporation) in addition to a variety of other tests, can help to address various questions (regarding, e.g., the presence of dementia, sequelae of head injury, and the patient's functional abilities). The likelihood of authorization is further increased when referrals are received from physicians who are unable to make a definitive medical diagnosis without additional neuropsychological data.

Referrals for assessment of attention deficit hyperactivity disorder are also quite common and, in more complicated cases, are likely to receive approval from the MCO. Some managed care companies currently include psychological assessment as part of the diagnostic protocol for attention deficit hyperactivity disorder (ADHD) and rely on some level of testing as a necessary component of diagnosis, beyond medical and educational evaluation. In addition to traditional measures of cognitive functioning, behavior rating scales such as the Achenbach Child Behavior Checklist (Achenbach & Edelbrock, 1983) and Conners Ratings Scales (Psychological Assessment Resources

[PAR], 1997) can be very cost-effective tools in shedding light on the presenting problem. Additionally, some psychologists use computer- based continuous performance tests to assess concentration and distractibility in their patients. Some of the research on these procedures, however, suggests caution in their use in diagnosis (Matier-Sharma, Perachio, Newcorn, & Sharma, 1995). Although it is unlikely that full batteries assessing intellectual, achievement, and personality factors will be routinely approved for initial evaluation of ADHD, more difficult cases that have been refractory to treatment may be viewed more favorably as appropriate for extensive workups. Despite the fact that assessment of ADHD often involves school functioning and cognitive evaluation, MCOs generally disallow testing for learning disabilities and educational placement, both of which are seen as the responsibility of the school system and are not deemed medically necessary.

Traditional psychological testing batteries, which involve comprehensive cognitive and personality evaluation, are more likely to be approved for seriously and persistently mentally ill patients, many of whom tend to be hospitalized repeatedly with complex and confusing clinical presentations. Many of these patients have proven refractory to outpatient psychiatric care, most of them have not responded to first line psychotherapeutic and somatic therapies, and diagnostic clarification is frequently requested by the admitting physician. Referral questions often involve questions of underlying character pathology, substance abuse, or organic involvement. It is important to note that this level of testing typically is approved only after the patient has undergone previous treatment that has been unsuccessful. It is interesting to speculate that a more complete psychological evaluation at the inception of such a course of treatment might have actually identified the problems earlier and ultimately reduced the overall cost of care. A more complete discussion of the role of testing in reducing treatment length is presented later in this chapter.

Although these traditional areas of testing may be available in order to add value to the benefit package in a typical MCO, routine approval in any single case should not be expected. Authorizations are, in part, a function of the background and sophistication of the case manager, and of the competence of the psychologist in the area of assessment requested and in the relationship between the case manager and the practitioner. Psychologists increase their chance of success in this regard by developing an ongoing and collegial partnership with the case manager. Providing information and benefits of testing in a particular case, educating the nonpsychologist case manager about testing, and presenting relevant information and the rationale for testing in nontechnical terms all increase the chances that authorizations are granted. Although empirical literature is not available to support the reality of testing benefits, psychologists have the opportunity over time to prove to the MCO the efficacy of their evaluations in terms of quality of care and cost on a case-by-case basis. The difficulty of the sell may be lessened in the traditional testing areas previously discussed as compared to others in which the added value of assessment is less widely appreciated. One of these areas involves the role of testing in reducing the length of treatment.

THE ROLE OF PSYCHOLOGICAL TESTING IN REDUCING THE LENGTH OF TREATMENT

No issue in managed mental health care has received more attention than that of reducing the length of treatment in both in- and outpatient settings. Long-term, intensive psychotherapy is discouraged and rarely authorized. Brief inpatient stays of 3 to 10 days and two to four outpatient visits per authorization are provided by MCO staff, who must review written treatment updates and/or require telephone consultation in order to approve further treatment. A common philosophy in MCOs involves what has been labeled "intermittent psychotherapy throughout the life cycle" (Cummings & Sayama, 1995), which emphasizes brief, focused intervention aimed at reduction of acute stress and restabilization at premorbid levels of functioning. Whereas this approach is highly appropriate for many patients presenting for treatment, it has significant limitations for the more seriously and persistently mentally disabled (Gabbard, 1994). MCOs often have attempted to apply their treatment philosophy across the board, without assessing the unique characteristics of patients, their problems, and the chronicity of their illnesses.

In response to the demands for brief, presumably cost-effective treatments, a great deal of attention has been directed to the development of models of therapy that promise to address patient difficulties in a time-limited and efficient manner (Budman & Gurman, 1988; Cummings & Sayama, 1995; Strupp & Binder, 1984). Although models differ and represent a variety of theoretical frameworks, including cognitive, behavioral, or dynamic, all have in common a search for a focus that informs treatment planning and establishes some well-circumscribed area to be addressed within a relatively short period of time. It follows, then, that careful evaluation and accurate diagnosis is necessary to ensure the appropriate selection of such highly focused, targeted treatment interventions. Psychologists therefore can begin to justify to the MCO the importance thorough pretreatment evaluation.

The identification of a treatment focus must be predicated on sound, comprehensive evaluation. Rather than eliminating or severely reducing pretreatment assessment, brief, targeted models of treatment require the practitioner to accumulate as much information as possible with regard to the patient's personality functioning, symptom picture, and risk factors, including suicidal potential and openness to treatment. An initial clinical interview rarely provides a clear, independent appraisal of all relevant problem areas or the patient's capacity to manage them effectively. Substance abuse problems, medical/organic influences, and characterological influences significantly affect treatment length by derailing therapy when the focus of the intervention is on another self-reported, and less relevant, problem. It is true that skillful clinicians ultimately uncover many of these more subtle problems and treatment resistances given enough time with the patient. A time-limited four to eight session course of treatment, however, often does not provide that opportunity. Paradoxically, efforts to eliminate unnecessary pretreatment assessment may result in protracted, inappropriate, and often unsuccessful treatment and ultimately higher costs to the MCO.

Although psychologists should be encouraged to advocate for more thorough pretreatment evaluation for their patients, the use of comprehensive and expensive batteries is often unnecessary and is likely to meet with disapproval from the case manager. Objective personality instruments, components of more comprehensive cognitive tests, and brief rating scales provide very useful and relevant information with regard to patient functioning, at relatively little cost in time and money.

The Minnesota Multiphasic Personality Inventory-2 (National Computer Systems [NCS], 1998), the Millon Clinical Multiaxial Inventory-III (NCS), the Symptom Check List-90-Revised (Derogatis, 1977), the Beck scales for depression and anxiety (Psychological Corporation, 1998), and subtests of the Wechsler scales can all be helpful in efficiently assessing and prioritizing problem areas in terms of severity and treatability. All of these assist in quickly establishing a treatment focus.

In order to meet their overall goals, MCOs cannot afford to sacrifice treatment quality simply to ensure a reduced length of care. Whereas the issues of treatment length and quality are inextricably linked, the role of psychological testing in ensuring quality of care and positive treatment outcomes within a model of time sensitive therapy is a critical one.

THE ROLE OF PSYCHOLOGICAL TESTING IN ENHANCING TREATMENT QUALITY AND OUTCOME

In recent years practitioners have responded to the call for brief, time-limited interventions by modifying their standard therapeutic approaches and offering a plethora of hybrid therapies aimed at quick problem resolution. Beutler (1991), Clarkin and Hurt (1988), and others have noted the proliferation of treatment approaches, most of which are based on the clinicians' experience and training rather than on the proven effectiveness of such approaches. Although this state of affairs has existed in the field historically, managed care has framed the problem in financial terms, insisting on documentation of treatment effectiveness and quality in order to justify expenditure of limited health care dollars.

A related development in the evolution of brief treatment is the creation of manualized therapies that delineate the parameters of treatment in terms of foci, techniques, and number of sessions (Beutler & Clarkin, 1990; Lambert & Bergin, 1994). To assess the quality and empirical foundation of many of these therapies, the American Psychological Association Task Force on Promotion and Dissemination of Psychological Procedures (1995) published a list of empirically supported treatments that met criteria for effectiveness and in the future, are likely to be viewed positively by MCOs.

Although the managed care industry may look favorably on the empirically based, manualized approaches to treatment, Harwood and his colleagues (Harwood et al., 1997) point out two major problems in using these highly standardized procedures. First, they note that most clinicians are unlikely to adhere in practice to the highly specific procedures developed in the clinical laboratory and will simply label their own approaches with the correct buzzwords in order to satisfy the MCO. Second, they note that these manuals are quite rigid in the application of treatment; are usually informed by a single theoretical orientation; and ignore the unique characteristics, dynamics, symptoms and response styles of individual patients. In order to avoid a packaged approach to treatment, several researchers discourage the inflexible use of a single manual and advocate a prescriptive approach to treatment selection. Here, treatment procedures independent of theory can be integrated, and nondiagnostic aspects of patients including cognitive ability, attitude and openness toward therapy, coping styles, and environmental contextual variables can be considered in treatment selection (Beutler, 1983; Beutler & Clarkin, 1990; Beutler & Harwood, 1995). Psychological testing and evaluation have the potential to accurately assess those patient dimensions apart from diagnosis in order to facilitate the appropriate matching of patients to both the therapist and the treatment approach. Advocation of testing in this area is likely to result in the efficiency and effectiveness that the managed mental health care industry endorses. A thorough presentation of this literature represented by what Norcross (1994) terms "prescriptive eclectic therapy" and what Beutler and Clarkin (1990) refer to as "systematic treatment selection" is well beyond the purpose of this chapter. However, a brief review of some of the representative patient dimensions identified for use in treatment selection and some proposed psychological instruments with which to measure them are presented in what follows.

Assessing Openness to Psychological Treatment

A patient's willingness to engage in psychological treatment and to be open to the therapy process is central to successful treatment outcome. Pretreatment evaluation of this openness assists in deciding which treatment, if any, is likely to be effective. Objective personality instruments, particularly the MMPI-2 (Butcher, 1990), are cost-effective measures designed to shed light on the issues of treatment readiness and patient expectations. The MMPI-2 validity scales as well as clinical, content, and supplementary scales can be used to evaluate a patient's willingness to view their problems as psychologically based, to engage in the therapeutic process, and to be open to change. For instance, patients who omit many questions on the MMPI-2 Cannot Say score (?) are unlikely to be cooperative in treatment and may be unwilling to discuss their difficulties. The Lie scale (L) and the K scale both measure defensiveness in the patient and reluctance to acknowledge psychological difficulties. Patients with significant elevations on both scales are seen as rigid, psychologically unsophisticated individuals who view themselves as emotionally fine and are typically poor candidates for therapy. The F scale reflects the degree of overall subjective distress the patient is reporting. When the score reaches a moderate elevation, this suggests that the patient is feeling enough discomfort to seek and be motivated for treatment. Excessively high or very low scores are often contraindicative of successful treatment because the patient is reporting either no problems (low score) or such emotional disorganization that short-term interventions would not be effective. Interpretation of MMPI-2 validity scores is a complicated task and requires the evaluation of a number of factors. In general, however, good candidates for psychological treatment who are willing to discuss their problems receive moderately elevated F scales in conjunction with low scores on L and K.

In addition to using MMPI-2 validity scales in assessing appropriate candidates for treatment, the instrument has several clinical and content scales which are useful to the practitioner faced with making cost-effective treatment decisions in the age of managed care. Significant elevations on Scale 1 (Hypochondriasis) and Scale 3 (Hysteria) suggest a preoccupation with physical complaints, the tendency to look for medical explanations for problems, and a lack of psychological mindedness. These characteristics augur poorly for positive treatment outcome, especially in traditional talk therapy, and often lead to noncompliance and premature termination (Butcher, 1990). On the other hand, elevations on Scale 2 (Depression) and Scale 7 (Psychasthenia) suggest that the patient is experiencing significant turmoil, including depression and anxiety, which motivates him or her to participate fully in treatment. When elevations on Scale 7 become extremely high, however, the patient is likely to become so bogged down in debilitating rumination that therapy can be difficult and slow. In order to limit treatment length, psychologists can utilize this information to establish a clear focus for treatment and to carefully select treatments that will not reinforce this ruminative behavior. Finally, MMPI-2 content scales, including the Negative Treatment Indicators scale and Negative Work Attitudes scale, are useful in assessing the patient's willingness to cooperate in treatment, to trust the therapist, and to mobilize the emotional resources to change. High scores on these scales are contraindicative of successful outcomes in psychotherapy.

Although practitioners are unlikely simply to terminate patients with a configuration of scores described above, the former should consider these data in selecting the most appropriate and time sensitive treatments for such patients given their measured expectations and predispositions.

Assessing Resistance Potential and Coping Style

Resistance, or what social psychologists call "reactance," involves a patient trait or state that results in sensitivity and opposition to the influence of others.

Beutler and his colleagues (Beutler, et al., 1991a; Beutler, Machado, Engle, & MacDonald, 1991b) found that therapy patients evaluated as possessing a high potential for resisting external influence had more positive treatment outcomes with nonauthoritative, nondirective approaches to therapy than with more directive approaches. The same researchers found the latter more successful with patients evaluated as possessing low levels of resistance and defensiveness. Thus, client-centered, supportive, and paradoxical interventions may be more effective with high-reactance patients, whereas approaches that focus on behavioral and cognitive therapy are more successful with patients who possess low levels of resistant defensiveness (Beutler, Sandowicz, Fisher, & Albanese, 1996). Beutler et al. (1991a) also demonstrated that this differential treatment response characterized patients who were evaluated as impulsive, aggressive, and antisocial. These individuals had better treatment outcomes when they received cognitive–behavioral interventions, whereas those found to be low in these personality characteristics responded more favorably to insight-oriented approaches.

Another dimension related to reactance is coping style, which is characterized as a set of personality and behavioral variables that determine how a patient deals with interpersonal conflicts and manages stress. Norcross and Beutler (1997) cite a number of studies that evaluate differential therapy outcome as a function of coping styles of the patient. Beutler and Clarkin (1990) describe an externalizer–internalizer patient dimension in which externalizers are conceived as outgoing, nurturance seeking, and prone to using acting out as a defense, and internalizers are described as introverted, constricted, and given to utilizing projection and intellectualization to manage stress. Beutler et al. (1991b) found that high externalizers responded best to behavioral treatment, whereas low externalizers had better outcomes with more insight-oriented approaches.

Assessment of coping style as well as resistant defensiveness with appropriate and inexpensive psychological testing can inform the practitioner about treatment selection as well as the degree of therapeutic intensity that will impact most favorably on treatment outcome. Pretreatment evaluation of these dimensions can reduce treatment length and maximize outcome by tailoring the therapeutic approach to each patient's style and personality disposition.

The MMPI-2 is well equipped to provide very relevant information regarding these dispositions. Reactance is conceptually similar in some ways to openness to treatment and can also be tapped by the MMPI-2 validity scales, L and K, both of which reflect defensiveness and resistance to seeing oneself as psychologically distressed. Additionally, elevations on Scale 6 (Paranoia), Scale 4 (Psychopathic Deviate), and the Negative Treatment Indicator scale describe individuals who are rebellious, suspicious, and distrustful of interpersonal relationships, and tend to have negative attitudes toward mental health professionals. Another instrument the Therapeutic Reactance Scale, was designed by Dowd and his colleagues specifically to assess reactance potential (Dowd, Milne, & Wise, 1991).

Coping style, particularly that type described on the externalizing–internalizing continuum, also can be assessed with the MMPI-2. Externalizers tend to score high on Scale 4 (Psychopathic Deviate), Scale 9 (Hypomania), and Scale 3 (Hysteria). Patients who obtain elevations on these scales typically act out their conflicts, and are socially outgoing, gregarious, and energetic, but are ultimately self-centered, dependent, and angry. Internalizers, on the other hand, receive elevated scores, particularly on Scale 2 (Depression), Scale 7 (Psychasthenia), and Scale 0 (Social Introversion–Extroversion); they are characterized as anxious, guilt ridden, and introverted, and handle their conflicts through intellectualization and undoing.

Assessing Problem Severity

Independent of patient diagnosis, personality and coping styles, and openness to treatment, the severity of the identified psychological problems can provide the managed care provider with valuable information regarding potential duration, intensity, and selection of treatment. Several researchers have found that in the treatment of depression, for instance, medication was more effective than psychotherapy for patients with moderate to severe clinical ratings of depression, whereas interpersonal psychotherapy was more effective for patients rated with mild to moderate levels of depression (Sotsky et al., 1991; Klerman, Weissman, Rounsaville, & Chevron, 1984). Managed care companies pay close attention to ratings of severity, or "level of functioning," in authorizing treatment visits and justifying ongoing contact with the provider. Several low-cost measurement devices rated both by the clinician and the patient are available, ranging from DSM-IV's Global Assessment of Functioning (American Psychiatric Association, 1994) to more sophisticated and psychometrically sound scales. The Beck Depression Inventory, the Beck Anxiety Inventory, the Hamilton Rating Scale for Depression (PAR, 1997), the Symptom Check List-90-Revised, and the Brief Symptom Index (NCS, 1998) all provide information on severity of psychiatric symptoms that can be administered early in treatment and readministered periodically to evaluate therapy progress and outcome.

THE ROLE OF PSYCHOLOGICAL TESTING AND EVALUATION IN PRIMARY CARE SETTINGS

MCOs, specifically health maintenance organizations, frequently rely on the primary care physician to triage all patients independent of their medical problems or symptoms. These physicians are faced with making treatment decisions that reflect both the financial and quality assurance philosophies mandated by their MCOs. Often faced with high patient volume, primary care providers (PCPs) have little time to evaluate the contribution of psychological and emotional factors to their patients' complaints, despite the fact that undiagnosed psychiatric problems may account for between 30% and 80% of all cases seen in primary care settings (Kelleher, 1995). The financial and emotional costs of missed or incomplete psychiatric diagnoses and comorbid psychological problems are considerable, especially in light of managed care's goal of reducing the overutilization of limited resources. Psychologists who can consult effectively with physicians and become a part of the health care team make a valuable contribution by providing appropriate evaluation and testing to patients in primary care settings.

It is well documented that psychological disorders significantly increase overall health care costs and negatively affect the economy in general (Kaplan, Sallis, & Patterson, 1993; Price & Cisco, 1985). Psychiatric and chemical dependency problems have a major impact on affected employees, who experience increases in the occurrence of accidents and in the amount of sick time needed as well as legal problems that result from violence and impaired judgment stemming from untreated disorders such as depression, anxiety, and alcoholism. Regier, Narrow, and Rae (1993) estimate that one third of Americans have experienced such disorders without treatment. The cost to employers, the government, and health care payers for the medical and criminal management of psychiatric and substance problems and their complications is astounding. In keeping with managed care's goal of effective utilization of resources, early and accurate assessment and referral of these problems can result in a marked reduction in health care costs. The addressing of these behavioral health problems despite their additional cost leads to significant savings in general health care, is referred to as the "medical cost offset" (American Psychological Association Practice Directorate, 1994). MCOs have a vested interest in identifying these disorders, and psychologists can contribute significantly in this endeavor.

One of the most obvious areas for psychological consultation and assessment involves assisting the physician in identification of psychological problems that mimic or complicate the treatment of organic illnesses. Depression, the "common cold of psychiatric illness," and anxiety both accompany and complicate the diagnosis of numerous medical conditions. Depression is a common sequela of stroke and several dementing illnesses. The diagnosis of a 75-year-old patient who presents with cognitive confusion, impaired memory, poor concentration, and "personality changes" as having irreversible dementia ignores the possibility that the patient might have a major depressive disorder (pseudodementia). Without adequate psychological assessment, this patient might not receive necessary treatment, which would address or at least ameliorate his or her condition. The confusing clinical picture that results from disorders such as chronic fatigue syndrome, lupus, thyroid conditions, and even the side effects of many drugs may be clarified by assessing independently for depressive and anxiety disorders, and treating the patient accordingly. Psychologists in their own practices must be aware of these disorders so they, too, can make appropriate referrals to their medical colleagues. The MMPI-2, as well as briefer rating scales (Hamilton Rating Scale for Depression; Beck Depression and Anxiety Scales; SCL-90-R), contains scales that measure depression and anxiety, and can be helpful in medical as well as mental health settings.

Even though psychological impairments such as depression or anxiety are not mimicking a true organic condition, PCPs must consider the role of these factors in a variety of illnesses including heart disease, cancer, diabetes, and gastrointestinal disorders as well as other stress-mediated and traumatic illnesses. Failure to diagnose the presence of psychological disorders in these cases not only ignores the emotional pain of the patient, but can risk compromising the patient's compliance with medical treatment. The instruments previously described, as well as the Millon Behavioral Health Inventory (MBHI; NCS, 1998), can offer valuable information to the PCP about managing such patients. The MBHI is an instrument designed to assess a patient's coping style with respect to physical illness, identify psychosomatic complications, and provide clinical data that inform treatment decisions.

Psychological testing and evaluation can also be useful to the PCP who deals with patients who are chronic somatizers and who report poorly defined symptoms, including chronic pain for which no physical etiology can be found. Instruments such as the MMPI-2, as well as briefer rating scales previously mentioned, can assist in the diagnosis of hypochondrical, hysterical, and pain disorders that bring patients to their PCPs. Clinical elevations on MMPI-2 Scale 1 (Hypochondriasis) and Scale 3 (Hysteria) are often indications that patients are converting psychological pain into the somatic realm. Such presentations should further indicate to the physician that the patient may have a significant emotional overlay to any organic problems identified, that treatment outcome and compliance are likely to be negatively affected by those problems, and that such patients often receive much secondary gain from their symptoms, frequently becoming emotionally dependent on medical attention.

PCPs who are considering referring patients for surgery can also benefit from psychological testing and assessment. In fact, surgical specialists, especially those who conduct elective procedures, may even require psychological clearance to evaluate prognosis, postsurgical recovery problems, and medical compliance. Instruments such as the MMPI-2 and the Millon Inventories provide numerous scales and indices that may suggest poor postsurgical recovery, including problems previously addressed such as high levels of depression, medication abuse potential, or high likelihood of somatization and psychological dependency.

Alcohol and substance abuse, in general, complicate the presentation of a variety of medical problems and symptoms commonly encountered by PCPs. Quick and accurate screening for substance abuse eliminates unnecessary treatment, conserves valuable resources, and ensure that the substance use disorder is treated directly rather than masked by its physical manifestations. Stout (1997) quotes a document published by the Georgia Psychological Association in 1991, in which it is estimated that 25% to 40% of patients in general hospital beds are actually being treated for complications of alcoholism. The MMPI-2, in particular, has several scales to evaluate substance abuse, including the MacAndrew Scale—Revised, the Addiction Acknowledgment Scale, and the Addiction Potential Scale. Elevations on any of these scales alert the clinician to the possibility of substance abuse. Other self-report inventories that are specific to substance abuse and can be administered quickly and in a cost-effective manner are also available.

Managed care's goals of cost-effective utilization of clinical services and reduction of unnecessary medical treatment are significantly impacted by the problem of malingering. There has been a great deal of research and writing on this topic in forensic psychology as well as in psychological assessment (Rogers, 1988), which is well beyond the scope of this chapter. However, psychologists should be aware that they have the potential to make a great contribution to their medical colleagues and managed care payers by using psychological and neuropsychological indices to rule out deception and malingering in the primary care setting.

ROLE OF PSYCHOLOGICAL TESTING IN THE EVALUATION OF TREATMENT OUTCOMES

Documentation of the effectiveness of mental health treatment will become increasingly more important in the future, when more providers, offering different therapeutic modalities, compete for the health care dollar. Credentialing as a means to demonstrate competence may be less important in the future. MCOs will demand empirical validation in support of claims that the procedures they fund (treatment, as well as testing and evaluation) actually result in real gains for their subscribers. Among all mental health providers, psychologists are uniquely qualified to assist the managed health care industry in evaluation and testing procedures that facilitate outcomes management and address the overall goals of the managed care industry—in this case to ensure the efficient utilization of limited resources without sacrificing the quality and effectiveness of treatment and evaluation. In working with managed care to help develop an evaluation system, psychologists ultimately will advance their own cause and ensure the acceptance of their skills, including psychological assessment, within the industry.

The demonstrable gains required by managed care may be quite varied and include areas of symptom reduction, functional status, and quality of life, as well as patient satisfaction (Stout, 1997). Psychologists historically have designed studies that measure treatment outcome by utilizing a prepost design and incorporating a variety of instruments to measure relevant symptoms or behavior that were the target of treatment. Many of the instruments described in this chapter are useful for these studies, but many are quite long and may reduce client compliance. The MMPI-2, the MCMI-III, and many of the projective devices can be helpful, but are often time consuming, especially in larger studies conducted by the MCO. Stout recommends briefer, self-administered measures that can be scored quickly and often with the assistance of the computer. Some of the scales mentioned earlier, including the Symptom Check

List-90-R, BASIS-32 (Eisen, Grob, & Klien, 1986), and the Beck scales for depression and anxiety, can be helpful for outcome evaluation.

Finally, evaluation of functional status expands outcome assessment beyond just symptoms and addresses issues related to overall health and well-being, the impact of role and physical limitations on patients, and the evaluation of social and economic functioning. Although instruments can be quite sophisticated in measuring functional status, many managed care companies use DSM-IV Axis V, Global Assessment of Functioning, as a simple measure of this dimension.

Patient satisfaction with care is a very straightforward indication of treatment efficacy. Whereas researchers have long been skeptical of the validity of self-report (Rohland & Langbehn, 1997; Atkinson & Caldwell, 1997), the managed care industry has embraced this methodology as a way to receive direct feedback about the services that they underwrite. Stout (1997) encouraged companies to develop their own "homegrown" versions of the instruments and recommended the inclusion of questions that involve quality of support staff, convenience of location, satisfaction with all dimensions of care, perceptions of improvement in problems, and willingness to recommend the services to others. Psychologists can be very helpful in designing these instruments to measure patient satisfaction, ensuring the appropriate structure of the questions, as well as in evaluating the reliability and validity of the instruments.

Psychologists are encouraged to develop a program of outcome evaluation within their own private practice, inpatient, or clinic settings. By providing outcome and patient satisfaction data to managed care companies psychologists gain the additional credibility of empirical validation of their work, increase the chances for authorization of services they request for their patients, and enhance their ability to obtain contracts from MCOs. The providing of data that documents that the use of psychological testing reduced treatment length, resulted in the successful use of differential approaches with different types of patients, and improved patient satisfaction as a function of patients being more "understood" through testing will be critical in the future if psychological assessment is to play a major role in managed mental health care.

SUMMARY

In summary, the role of psychological evaluation and testing appears to be an important and valuable one within a managed care environment. Within a mental health environment they can assist in establishing a valid diagnosis early in treatment, crystallize a focus for brief treatment, enhance quality by effectively matching patients to treatment approaches, and reduce the length of treatment by assessing openness and attitudes toward therapy. Evaluation and testing also play a critical role in primary care settings where the need to rule out psychological problems and consider their role in treatment compliance is crucial to quality care and cost-effective utilization of services. To take advantage of such contributions, psychologists must help to reverse the general tendency within the managed care industry to limit or eliminate those very services. Psychologists must join with their managed care colleagues in finding ways to maximize their common goal of enhancing quality of care. Psychological practitioners must be willing to learn about the managed care environment—its philosophy and goals; must strive to educate the MCO about the value of testing, including how evaluation will impact on those goals; and must be conservative and discriminating whenever they request authorization for testing. Such a partnership undoubtedly will have a very beneficial effect on managed care's attitude toward testing and evaluation in the future.

REFERENCES

Achenbach, T. M., & Edelbrock, C. (1983). *Manual for the child behavior checklist and revised child behavior profile.* Burlington, VT: Authors.

American Psychiatric Association. (1994). *Diagnostic and statistical manual of mental disorders* (4th ed.). Washington, DC: Author.

American Psychological Association Clinical Division 12. (1993). What is clinical psychology? Oklahoma City, OK: Author.

American Psychological Association Practice Directorate. (1994). APA member focus groups on the health care environment: A summary report. Washington, DC: American Psychological Association.

American Psychological Association Task Force on Promotion and Dissemination of Psychological Procedures. (1995). Training in and dissemination of empirically-validated treatments: Report and recommendations. *Clinical Psychologist 48*(1), 3–23.

Atkinson, M. J., & Caldwell, L. (1997). The differential effects of mood on patients' ratings of life quality and satisfaction with their care. *Journal of Affective Disorders, 44,* 169–175.

Beutler, L. E. (1983). *Eclectic psychotherapy: A systematic approach.* New York: Pergamon.

Beutler, L. E. (1991). Have all won and must all have prizes? Revisiting Luborsky et al's verdict. *Journal of Consulting and Clinical Psychology 59,* 1–7.

Beutler, L. E., & Clarkin, J. F. (1990). *Systematic treatment selection: Toward targeted therapeutic interventions.* New York: Brunner/Mazel.

Beutler, L. E., Engle, D., Mohr, D. C., Daldrup, R. J., Bergan, J., Meredith, K., & Merry, W. (1991a). Predictors of differential response to cognitive, experiential, and self directed psychotherapeutic procedures. *Journal of Consulting and Clinical Psychology 59,* 333–340.

Beutler, L. E., & Harwood, T. M. (1995). Prescriptive psychotherapies. *Applied and Preventive Psychology 4,* 89–100.

Beutler, L. E., Machado, P. P., Engle, D., & MacDonald, R. (1991b). Differential patient x treatment maintenance of treatment effects among cognitive, experiential, and self-directed psychotherapies. *Journal of Psychotherapy Integration 3,* 15–31.

Beutler, L. E., Sandowicz, M., Fisher, D., & Albanese, A. L. (1996). Resistance in psychotherapy: What can be concluded from empirical research? *In Session: Psychotherapy in Practice, 2,* 77–86.

Budman, S. H., & Gurman, A. S. (1988). *Theory and practice of brief therapy.* New York: Guilford Press.

Butcher, J. N. (1990). *MMPI-2 in psychological treatment.* New York: Oxford University Press.

Clarkin, J. D., & Hurt, S. W. (1988). Psychological Assessment: Tests and rating scales. In J. A. Talbot, R. E. Hales, & S. C. Yudofsky (Eds.), *Textbook of psychiatry.* Washington, DC: American Psychiatric Press.

Cummings, N., & Sayama, M. (1995). *Focused psychotherapy: A casebook of brief, intermittent psychotherapy throughout the life cycle.* New York: Brunner/Mazel.

Derogatis, L. R. (1977). *Symptoms checklist-90-revised manual.* Baltimore, MD: Clinical Psychometric Research.

Dowd, E. T., Milne, C. R., & Wise, S. L. (1991). The therapeutic reactance scale: A measure of psychological reactance. *Journal of Counseling and Development 69,* 541–545.

Eisen, S., Grob, M., & Klien, A. (1986). BASIS: The development of a self-report measure for psychiatric evaluation. *Psychiatric Hospital, 6,* 165–171.

Gabbard, G. O. (1994). Inpatient services: The clinician's view. In R. K. Schreter, S. S. Sharstein, & C. A. Schreter (Eds.), *Allies and adversaries* (pp. 22–30). Washington, DC: American Psychiatric Press.

Golden, C. J., Hammeke, T. A., & Purisch, A. D. (1980). *The Luria Nebraska neuropsychological battery: Manual.* Los Angeles, CA: Western Psychological Services.

Harwood, T. M., Beutler, L. E., Fisher, D., Sandowicz, M., Albanese, A. L., & Baker, M. (1997). In Butcher, J. N. (Ed.), *Personality assessment in managed health care* (pp. 13–41). New York: Oxford University Press.

Kaplan, R. M., Sallis, J. F. Jr., & Patterson, T. L. (1993). *Health and human behavior.* New York: McGraw–Hill.

Kelleher, K. (1995). Mental health in primary care: Major trends and issues. *Policy in Perspective, 1,* 3–4.

Klerman, G. L., Weissman, M. M., Rounsaville, B. J., & Chevron, E. S. (1984). *Interpersonal psychotherapy of depression.* New York: Basic Books.

Klump, K., & Butcher, J. N. (1997). Psychological tests in treatment planning. In J. N. Butcher (Ed.), *Personality assessment in managed health care* (pp. 93–130). New York: Oxford University Press.

Lambert, M. L., & Bergin, A. E. (1994). The effectiveness of psychotherapy. In A. E. Bergin & S. L. Garfield (Eds.), *Handbook of psychotherapy and behavior change* (4th ed., pp. 72–113). New York: Wiley.

Matier-Sharma, K., Perachio, N., Newcorn, S. H., & Sharma, V. (1995). Differential diagnosis of adhd: Are objective measures of attention, impulsivity and activity level helpful? *Child Neuropsychology, 1,* 118–127.

National Computer Systems. (1998). *Product catalog.* Minnetonka, MN: Author.

Norcross, J. C. (1994). *Prescriptive eclectic therapy* [Videotape]. Videotape in the APA Psychotherapy Videotape Series. Washington, DC: American Psychological Association Books).

Norcross, J. C., & Beutler, L. E. (1997). Determining the therapeutic relationship of choice in brief therapy. In Butcher, J. N. (Ed.), *Personality Assessment in Managed Health Care* (pp. 13–41). New York, NY: Oxford University Press.

Price, D. P., & Cisco, A. (1985). The economic costs of alcohol and drug abuse and mental illness. *Medical Care, 23,* 109–111.

Psychological Assessment Resources. (1997). *Comprehensive catalog.* Odessa, FL: Author.

Psychological Corporation. (1998). *Product catalog.* San Antonio, TX: Author.

Regier, D. A., Narrow, W. E., & Rae, D. S. (1993). The defacto U.S. mental and addictive disorders service system: Epidemiologic catchment area perspective. *Archives of General Psychiatry, 50,* 85–94.

Reitan, R. M., & Wolfson, D. (1993). *The Halstead–Reitan neuropsychological battery: Theory and clinical interpretation* (2nd ed.). Tucson, AZ: Neuropsychological Press.

Resnick, R. J., & DeLeon, P. H. (1995). News from Washington, D.C. *Professional Psychology: Research and Practice 26,* 3–4.

Rogers, R. (Ed.) (1988). *Clinical assessment of malingering and deception.* New York: Guilford Press.

Rohland, B. M., & Langbehn, D. R. (1997). Characterizing quality of life among patients with chronic mental illness: A critical examination of the self-report methodology: Commentary. *American Journal of Psychiatry, 154,* 1478–1479.

Sotsky, S. M., Glass, D. R., Shea, T. M., Pilkonis, P. A., Collins, J. F., Elkin, I., Watkins, J. T., Imber, S. D., Leber, W. R., Moyer, J., & Oliveri, M. E. (1991). Patient predictors of response to psychotherapy and pharmacotherapy: Findings in the NIMH treatment of depression collaborative research program. *American Journal of Psychiatry 148,* 997–1008.

Stout, C. E. (1997). *Psychological assessment in managed care.* New York: Wiley.

Strupp, H. H., & Binder, J. L. (1984). *Psychotherapy in a new key.* New York: Basic Books.

3

Individual Psychotherapy and Managed Care

Carol S. Austad
Central Connecticut State University

The curtain has opened on an era of managed mental health care. Mental health providers find themselves increasingly accountable for the cost and effectiveness of their treatments and the satisfaction of patients and payers (Barlow, 1996; Cummings, & Sayana, 1995). Unlike psychotherapists of the late 1970s, psychotherapists today need to be keenly aware of how the economic milieu affects psychological practice. Psychotherapists are confronted with the challenge of incorporating the demands of payers into the way individual psychotherapy is delivered; if they cannot respond to this challenge, psychotherapists may be faced with a loss of finances, feelings of competency and personal satisfaction (Berlin, 1969; Hoyt, 1985). However, although change can be stressful, it can also be positive, providing new insights and previously unthought of opportunities (Bloom, 1997; Carter, 1993). Mental health practitioners must learn to navigate through the ever-changing waters of unfamiliar practice demands.

Faced with a health care revolution, psychotherapists have come face-to-face with the realization that health care delivery and psychotherapy are intricately interrelated. Although psychotherapists have a great need to know about the integration of financial, managerial, clinical, and preventive aspects of mental health care (Appelbaum, 1993), their education has given them little formal training in these areas (Austad, 1996a, 1996b; Bloom, 1990; Boaz, 1988). Although the practitioner psychologist is most immediately and directly affected by these changes, the trickle-down effect makes the evolution of American health care a matter of concern to all psychologists (Callan & Yeager, 1991). Changes in the practice of psychotherapy will influence academic, research, and, most important, education and training activities (Wilson, 1996).

A rapidly changing health care system calls for rapidly changing attitudes on the part of mental health professionals. Successful adaptation requires a restructuring of perspective, a flexibility of attitudes, and an intentional effort to perceive events differently (Austad, 1996b). At this historical crossroad, it is imperative for psychologists to open their minds and expand their consciousness, examining how their current professional attitudes will affect their practice in the future.

The purpose of this chapter is to stimulate thinking and promote discourse about how the reorganization of the mental health care environment is affecting the practice of individual psychotherapy. The following core issues are considered:

1. What factors in the present health care system affect the practice of psychotherapy?
2. What strategies of coping have been used by psychologists and other psychotherapists to adapt to managed care settings?
3. What are the characteristics of psychotherapies that fit into managed care settings?
4. What models of psychotherapy offer the greatest promise and serve the most people in a clinically effective and socially useful way?
5. What changes need to be made to the practice of psychotherapy and the training of psychotherapists in the current, ongoing, and future reorganization of health care?

PERSONAL EXPERIENCE

On a personal note, I would like to share how my own experience in a managed care environment altered my attitude and orientation about psychotherapy. I hope this will help the reader appreciate the remainder of this chapter.

I began my managed care therapy career in a federally funded, not-for-profit health maintenance organization (HMO). Within this environment, a mental health provider deals with a defined population of patients who receive all of their health services from the HMO. Therapy clients are a subset of the membership of the general health population insured by the HMO. Therapists are salaried employees.

I was a therapist with long-term psychodynamic training, but graduate school had not prepared me for working at the HMO. I learned on the job from experienced HMO clinicians. I soon realized that the HMO was a microcosm of the health care universe. Mental health staff had to care for all of the mental health needs of the membership, a situation that mirrored the social issues vexing all of American mental health care. Our mission was to provide psychotherapy to all of our membership in the most fair and equitable way, and our motto was, "Our patient is not just the single individual but the sociological matrix of the entire health plan membership." Mental health staff became creative in trying to balance their clinical resources, devising innovative ways of maintaining, improving, and repairing the mental health of the HMO members.

I soon became what I call a "temporal eclectic," learning that time was a resource and that I had none to waste. One day, I had a core realization. As my client load built up in my first year, I noticed that some clients did not return after one or two sessions. As a psychodynamically trained clinician, I assumed these no-returns represented treatment failures. Each caused me to doubt my therapeutic prowess. What did I do wrong? Why hadn't the patient returned?

I remember the day that Joyce came back to see me after an absence of 1 year. Until her visit, I assumed she had been a treatment failure. She had never responded to my follow up call inquiring if she wanted to reschedule. Then, a year later, I found myself sitting face-to-face with Joyce, who told me, "I got so much from our conversation a year ago, I wanted to see you again to get a jump start." Utterly amazed, I was jolted into a new perspective by her words. A truth was evident. What I had interpreted to be treatment failure—what my supervisors would have attributed to my lack of therapeutic sophistication—was actually a success. A one-time session could be a powerful introject for the patient. It was possible to have a very short-term intervention that yielded long-term positive effects. I saw Joyce from then on intermittently, when she felt it was necessary. I became aware of the great faith the therapist must have in patients' abilities to judge what they did and did not require.

More of these "Joyce-type" events occurred, causing me to revise my core concept of psychotherapy. I combed the literature and discovered that others shared my experiences. Nicholas Cummings, who had been chief psychologist at Kaiser in Northern California and founder of Biodyne, had already published a substantial amount on what I had discovered. He called it "intermittent psychotherapy throughout the life cycle."

Furthermore, as John O. Prochaska has written, people come to therapy in different states of readiness to change. In addition, I know from the results of my own studies that long-term therapists can work contentedly in some managed care environments provided that they assume a new perspective and make some appropriate attitudinal adjustments. The remainder of this chapter describes and discusses these issues.

MANAGED CARE AND ITS EFFECT ON PSYCHOTHERAPY

The recent rise of managed care in the United States is no accident. Economic conditions provided fertile soil and sowed the seeds that produced the blossoming of managed care (Austad & Hoyt, 1992; Castro, 1994; Starr, 1982). The inability of professionals to curb out-of-control costs is one reason that health care became an issue of political, economic, and social concern (Bergin, 1992; Koss & Butcher, 1986; Lambert, Shapiro, & Bergin, 1986). Managed care manufactured effective methods of managing costs and reducing health care cost inflation, such as monitoring and reviewing treatment, decreasing unnecessary hospital days and stays, eliminating many unnecessary procedures, and altering provider and patient fiscal incentives (Davis, 1990; Ellwood, 1988; Feldman, 1992).

Delivering the most cost-effective health care to the largest number of people has become a high priority since the early 1980s (Bennett, 1988; VandenBos, 1986). Payers (insurance companies, the government, employers, and individuals) want to finance health care benefits, which include necessary, effective treatment, while eliminating waste (Bowers & Knapp, 1993; Clemens, 1995). They continue to ask mental health professionals questions that beg to be answered. What type of psychotherapy performed by what type of professional therapist is most effective for the patients for whom we are paying medical benefits? Can outcomes data back up claims? As one CEO mentioned to me, "In short, how can the consumer, the patient, and the payer, (that's me, the employer) get the most bang for their bucks?

Thus, in the evolution of mental health care, only the diagnostic, preventive, and therapeutic treatments that prove to be effective on the basis of outcome are financed by insurers. Society determines which beneficial services to exclude and which to provide (Dacso & Dacso, 1995).

By holding the purse strings, managed care is a powerful force shaping contemporary psychotherapy practice (Cummings, Pallak, & Cummings, 1996). By underwriting specific types of psychotherapy, that is, by subscribing only to providers who offer eclectic psychotherapy, managed care influences providers to select models that are compatible with a short-term benefit design or to fail in their efforts to practice with managed care companies. The models of therapy that survive are those that can be used effectively within managed care settings, and the psychotherapists who endure are those who use such models with expertise. Those who do not are in danger of extinction.

THE PSYCHOTHERAPIST COPING WITH MANAGED CARE

Despite intense practitioner reactions to its unanticipated rise to dominance, the picture is clear; it is no longer possible to perform psychotherapy as if it were independent of its economic environment (England & Cole, 1993). Successful therapists will adapt to the demand characteristics (Goran, 1992). Therefore, graduate education and professional training must include information about adapting traditional practice to the managed care environment (Flinn, McMahon, & Collings, 1987).

Undoubtedly, therapists must cope with these abrupt changes and struggles, yet only a few researchers have attempted to study the feelings, attitudes, and thoughts of clinicians who have adapted their psychotherapy practice to managed care (Kohrman, 1986; Lange, Chandler-Guy, Forti, Foster-Moore, & Rohman, 1988). In a series of interview and survey studies, some investigators asked staff model managed care (a dying breed of managed care) therapists to describe how they fit their practice into a staff model managed care setting (Austad, 1992; Austad, Sherman, Morgan, & Holstein, 1992).

The majority of participants reported that they experienced culture shock on entering a managed care system. They learned on the job and adapted by using psychotherapy methods that were focused, goal directed, and short-term, with a view of the therapeutic relationship that emphasizes the notions of health and independence, and de-emphasizes pathology and dependence. The majority surveyed thought that a benefit package of 20 sessions per calendar year was adequate to treat most patients with good quality of care. Belief in, and use of, short-term therapy in lieu of longer term therapy was common. The number of therapists who used the psychodynamic model as their primary practice model dwindled while the number of therapists who ranked "eclectic" as their most frequently used model increased. Competence in short-term therapy and crisis management were highly valued skills. Therapists emphatically declared that graduate training did not prepare them for work in a managed care setting. Contemporary training methods are not preparing new therapists to practice in managed care settings, yet training and supportive interpersonal processes are highly valued in adapting to setting demands.

CORE CHARACTERISTICS OF GOOD MANAGED CARE PSYCHOTHERAPY

In 1988, I coined the phrase "HMO therapy," which I defined as psychotherapy conducted in not-for-profit HMOs with core characteristics (Austad, 1993; Austad and Berman, 1991; Austad & Hoyt, 1992; Austad, Kisch, & DeStefano, 1989; Bauer & Kobos, 1987; Bistline, Sheridan, & Winegar, 1991; Hoyt and Austad, 1992). The following features are essential to conducting high-quality, effective short-term therapy in good managed care settings.

1. Pragmatic Therapeutic Consumer Alliance

Research shows that a strong positive, therapeutic alliance and the patient's expectations of therapy account for a good percentage of change in therapy (Lambert, 1991). Therefore, the successful managed care therapist forms a solid therapeutic alliance as rapidly as possible by incorporating the reality of limited time and resources into the therapeutic work. The therapist encourages autonomy and independence rather than transference and dependence. In this teamlike alliance, elements of consumerism are openly acknowledged. The therapist is seen as more of a mental health consultant to the patient than as an authority figure, imbued with almost magical powers of curing the psyche. Patient and payer satisfaction are part of the criterion for success. Whereas in the past, therapist autonomy—either clinical or economic—was seldom challenged, the expectation today is that the therapist must be accountable to demonstrate the effectiveness of his/her interventions in helping the patient make necessary gains. Thus, the consumer elements of the therapy/patient relationship has given it much more of an aura of a consultation/business model rather than a unique, enigmatic, mystical relationship with an end goal of restructuring character.

With the role of "doctor of the soul" changed to that of health care/business consultant, a homogenation of the therapy professions is occurring. Whereas traditionally, some professions claimed to be better than others at conducting psychotherapy by virtue of superior training and status, the current trend is to recompense for service according to diagnostic code, not provider training (Stein, 1994). "Equal pay for equal work" means that professions are competing for the right to perform psychotherapy. Because no substantial evidence shows that one profession can perform psychotherapy better than another (Dawes, 1994; Lambert, 1991; Seligman, 1995), such homogenization results from payers wanting assurance that treatment decisions are intended to enhance patient welfare and not provider income (Spencer, Frank, & McGuire, 1996).

2. Active Positive Therapist

The therapist is authoritative about mental health issues, but not authoritarian. In the role of expert, mental health consultant, the therapist is less likely to pathologize the patient's condition and more likely to emphasize the building of patient strengths. The therapist is active, fostering positivity and potency within the client. Structuring therapeutic contacts, the therapist recommends alternative interventions for the patient. The therapist involves significant others in the therapy process as needed.

3. Focused Assessment

Rapid, accurate assessment of patient needs occurs in the here and now. The therapist responds as rapidly as possible to the demands of people in the real world. He or she evaluates and selects which interventions are necessary and sufficient to develop and execute an effective, efficient treatment plan. The therapist is eclectic, is not bogged down in theoretical constructs, and is willing to accept what the patient says at face value and work with salient issues. The therapist does not interpret its meaning at a level that delays taking helpful action immediately.

4. Outcomes-Based, Functional, Treatment Goals

The therapist clearly defines his/her role in the life of the patient and acts as a mental health advisor, prepared to offer up-to-date, empirically based treatments for the patient. The managed care milieu underwrites treatment goals that emphasize everyday adaptation to the stresses of life as well as functional goals such as adjustments to work, school, and interpersonal tasks. Insight and personal growth are not highly valued as goals in themselves, as they were in traditional psychoanalytic models. A contract for specific, achievable goals is negotiated. The scheduling of sessions and the duration of treatment are agreed on by both. The responsibilities of patient and therapist are clearly articulated. The patient's assignments include, at minimum, bringing relevant material to the sessions, cooperating in extra session assignments, and implementing behavioral change outside of therapeutic meetings.

5. Rapid Response to Need/Crisis Intervention Preparedness

Prompt handling of emergencies is highly valued. The therapist assumes that early access to psychotherapy can avoid the intensification of clinical problems and symptoms, and decreases the risk of overintensive therapeutic involvement.

6. Parsimonious and Flexible Use of Interventions

The therapist's preferred method of intervention is that which is least extensive, least expensive, and least intrusive. Group therapy, psychoeducation, community resources, family intervention, and self-help groups are important forms of treatment and are not merely adjunctive aids to individual therapy. The therapist respects and recommends alternative treatment approaches such as self-help groups and psychoeducation. The schedule of therapy—frequency, length, and timing—is as cost effective as possible.

7. Discrimination Between Medically Necessary and Discretionary Psychotherapy

Much as plastic surgeons distinguish between essential reconstructive surgery and cosmetic plastic surgery, therapists in tune with managed care are able to separate medically necessary psychotherapy from discretionary psychotherapy. Necessary care is considered a health entitlement and therefore should be funded by the payers. Discretionary psychotherapy, on the other hand, is not essential to mental health and ought to be funded by the person receiving treatment.

8. Temporal Eclecticism

The temporally eclectic therapist possesses the ability to work in both long- and short-term modalities, as well as the wisdom to know when to apply each method (Austad, 1996b). Such therapists believe that claims made about temporal standards need to have some empirical base. It is important for psychotherapy time guidelines to be data driven. For example, a psychotherapist who insists, despite a lack of empirically based guidelines for temporal dimensions of treatment, that a patient needs 200 sessions stands on shaky ground.

Temporally eclectic psychotherapists question some basic assumptions held by traditional therapists. The former believe that long-term bias—a partiality to favor long-term therapy despite the lack of any substantial data to support such preference—has permeated practice until recently. They also point out that psychoanalysis is not necessarily the best form of therapy. No definitive empirical evidence exists to demonstrate that long-term psychotherapy is superior to short-term psychotherapy (Hoyt, 1985).

Temporal eclectics point out that most therapy actually practiced in the United States is brief. Additionally, brief work, or therapy that is short by design rather than by default, can be extremely effective. Data suggest that the overwhelming majority of psychotherapy cases are brief; that more people can be reached, served, and helped by short-term therapy; and that for many clients, brief treatment not only is effective but is all that is required (Howard, Davidson, Mahoney, Orlinsky, & Brown, 1989; Levin, 1992; Olson & Pincus, 1994; Phillips, 1985). Temporal eclectics believe that therapists need to be aware of the "clinician's illusion" that all therapy is long term (Cohen & Cohen, 1984). Patients in long-term therapies represent only a small percentage of those who seek therapy and are not truly representative of most patients.

Temporally eclectic therapists know that there are always some people who need long-term mental health assistance, but long-term care does not necessarily mean long-term traditional therapy. Like elective cosmetic surgery, long-term therapy with increased insight into one's own psychological complexities as the primary outcome cannot be classified as "medically necessary." However, if an individual is disabled and in need of care, or finds long-term therapy medically necessary, then it is available to the patient just as chemotherapy is accessible to the cancer patient. Discretionary therapy, a wonderful personal growth experience, should be financed out-of-pocket by the individual seeking treatment (Austad & Hoyt, 1992).

9. Developmental Orientation

The managed care therapist views a human being from a holistic, life-span development perspective. Every person is a life in progress. The therapist realizes that people are most likely to seek out psychotherapy when they experience increased levels of stress.

10. Psychological Family Doctor or Primary Care Orientation

Once a solid psychotherapeutic relationship is established, the psychotherapeutic dyad is seen as a continuous, intermittent interaction between therapist and patient that can extend throughout the life cycle. The psychotherapist is the psychological family doctor. Patients seek out treatment, or consultation with the mental health provider, when they need care and stop treatment when the therapy consultation is completed. Thus, contact between therapist and patient is carried out as needed in brief episodes over the life span through a succession of interrupted installments (Cummings, 1986).

11. Medical/Nonmedical Collaboration

The managed care non-medical mental health provider relates to multiple types of medical providers. Behavioral medicine and psychopharmacology are areas in which the nonmedical provider must intervene in order to use effective psychotherapeutic interventions. First, the integration of behavioral and biomedical science has led to the increasing need to apply behavior modification methods to the enhancement of prevention, diagnosis, treatment, and rehabilitation. Mental health professionals are now frequently asked to use psychotherapeutic interventions to help medical patients comply with treatment, adjust to medical conditions, and cope with disability and death. As mental health care becomes more fully integrated into general health care, behavioral techniques that enhance health-related problems will play an even more significant role in producing effective psychotherapy.

Second, communication with both primary care physicians and psychiatrists is essential to the integration of psychopharmacology and psychotherapy. Whether the therapist works in a staff model setting where it is easy to interact with primary care physicians or in a mental health group practice where contact is less likely and accessible, liasoning between the medical doctor and the primary care physician can only enhance the patient's treatment by treating the patient with a more holistic approach.

12. Willingness for Review and Evaluation

Because the managed care therapist is committed to delivering cost-effective therapy, data and feedback about practice habits are welcomed. The therapist is willing to participate in quality assurance reviews and also conducts outcome research or participates in global management information systems. He or she recognizes that quality, cost, and utilization management are linked. The development of adequate management information systems to assess the outcomes of the therapists' practices is considered to be an integral part of delivering care. Therapists believe that outcome measurements and use of data to document their own performance and appropriateness of procedures is commendable (Rodriguez, 1994).

13. Outpatient Versus Inpatient Treatment Orientation

Because it is seen as maximally intrusive, inpatient status is the court of last resort and all efforts are made to maintain the patient in an outpatient capacity. The belief is strong that a less restrictive environment is preferable to an overly intrusive one, and there is recognition that hospitalization can produce iatrogenic effects.

14. Current Knowledge About Research

The need for research designed to support decision making in the delivery of mental health services is recognized and highly valued (Fonagy & Target, 1996; Newman & Tejeda, 1996). The good managed care therapist knows that the scientific method is a self-critical approach essential to practicing high-quality psychotherapy in an applied setting. His or her breadth of knowledge of the recent empirical data base is deep enough to guide him- or herself in choosing the most desirable therapeutic interventions.

15. Revised Ethical Thinking

A new health care environment has produced new ethical dilemmas. Therapists who work in managed care settings know that it is necessary to envision a professional code of ethics as an organic entity that may be revised to guide practitioners in an ever-changing health care system (Olsen, 1995; Sabin, 1994a, 1994b; Webb, Rothschild, Monroe, 1994). Managed care practitioners are faced with a number of ethical concerns, including issues around quality, quantity, and continuity of care; patient freedom of choice; third-party intrusion into therapy; patient abandonment; the application of appropriate guidelines, outcome measures, and utilization review; confidentiality; provider autonomy; truth in advertising; and working with underprivileged groups. Furthermore, there is an obvious need for psychotherapists to articulate a clear-cut social ethic that assures fair and equal access to needed therapy for all members of the population. Professional organizations need to keep abreast of ethical dilemmas and monitor problems (Austad, Hunter, & Morgan, 1998; Austad & Sheridan, 1992).

These 15 core characteristics that are valued by high-quality managed care therapists show that psychotherapy and the role of the therapist and patient are continually evolving. The changes are not attributable to managed care alone, but managed care has acted as a catalyst by exerting pressure on mental health professionals to deliver specific types of services, and by altering the overall view of what constitutes appropriate treatment.

MODELS TO HELP THE MOST PEOPLE

Models of psychotherapy that contain the 15 core characteristics described above are likely to survive and thrive. With over 400 therapy models in existence today (Bauer & Kobos, 1987; Kleinke, 1994), practitioners may have difficulty selecting appropriate treatments. The following review briefly describes psychotherapy models that have been developed, implemented, or have potential for successful use in managed care settings. Thus far the effectiveness of these models and their methods is not as grounded in empirical data as it should be. Research shows that the superiority of one form of therapy over another has not been clearly established. The current research shows that psychotherapy itself is effective and more extensive outcome studies need to be conducted. Therapists are now exploring how to conceptualize therapy in a way that is most integrative and that can synthesize various discrepant models.

Intermittent Brief Therapy Throughout the Life Cycle: The New Paradigm

The intermittent brief psychotherapy throughout the life cycle model was devised by Nicholas Cummings, chief psychologist at Kaiser Permanente of northern California, a managed care setting (Cummings, 1991a, 1991b; Cummings & Sayana, 1995). At the same time that Cummings developed his therapy, Michael Bennett (1984), at Harvard Health Plan, developed his own version of intermittent therapy. This simple but comprehensive model constitutes a new paradigm for the conduct of modern day psychotherapy. Although many short-term therapy systems provide insights, methods, and techniques to help a person cope with life's difficulties, they lack comprehensiveness and continuity of care, providing piecemeal help. Methods for treating specific patient populations with specific problems at specific times in life are needed. The intermittent model can serve as a conceptual umbrella under which other models of psychotherapy can be subsumed, organized, and integrated. Intermittent therapy is based on a life-span view of human development and pragmatic altruism. It represents a paradigm shift in that it moves away from the traditional views that individual psychotherapy must be lengthy, all-encompassing, and conducted in weekly meetings. The concept of psychological cure is replaced with a notion of psychological intervention or consultation that serves as a catalyst in helping patients attain their attain their best psychological adjustment. Most importantly, this model values focused therapeutic work and changes the role of the therapist from expert authority figure to expert consultant. This is culturally relevant because it views psychotherapy in a way that is compatible with our knowledge base about how people change, and with the economic and social pressures facing Americans today.

Whereas in the more traditional, psychoanalytic models, therapy has a discrete beginning, middle, and end, based on an artificial schema of how human relationships work, intermittent psychotherapy provides a framework for the conduct of long-term psychotherapy in which patients receive long-term care rather than long-term treatment. The patient is viewed as a human being who grows, develops, and changes throughout his or her entire life cycle. A part of normal life is to encounter a variety of problems with work, relationships, finances, health, and the like. Furthermore, life contains a series of typical and predictable developmental tasks and junctures. Crises typically arise when a person is negotiating developmental junctures or milestones such as entering adolescence, adulthood, marriage, parenthood, midlife, and old age; facing inevitable losses; and ultimately confronting one's own death. The individual may need assistance from a therapist as a consultant to help him or her to negotiate changes. Anxiety often accompanies these stressors. The ability to resolve developmental difficulties and problems of living can be hampered if this anxiety is too great and the patient regresses, using maladaptive ways of coping that were used and learned earlier in life. A therapist or mental health consultant can render treatments that help the patient to secure more adaptive ways of coping and negotiating their own psychological well being. The emphasis in this therapy is on treating the pitfalls of normal human development realistically, pragmatically, efficiently, and effectively through a variety of techniques.

The therapist assumes the role of "psychological family doctor," which is analogous to that of the family medical doctor. The therapist adheres to a patient's bill of rights. The guiding principle of such treatment asserts that a patient is entitled to relief from pain, anxiety, and depression in the shortest time possible with the least amount of intrusion into his or her psyche as is necessary. The therapist–patient contract holds that the therapist will never ask the patient to do anything until the patient is ready to do it, and the therapist will never abandon the patient as long as the patient needs the therapist. In return for such therapist behavior, the patient is obligated to make the therapist obsolete as soon as he or she possibly can.

Cummings (1991a) also devised his own unique way of categorizing patients and problems. His methods include an operational diagnosis (why the patient came in today), an implicit contract (unconscious motivation and resistance), and an explicit therapeutic contract. Rather than depend upon DSM-IV formal diagnosing, he uses four questions to structure each discrete episode of treatment: Who is presenting? Why now? What for? And How? He categorizes patients into those who are analyzable (onions) and those who are not analyzable (garlic). "Onions" are clients with anxiety disorders, phobias, depression, hysteria and conversion neurosis, and obsessive–compulsive personality disorders. "Garlics" are clients with addictions, personality disorders, impulse disorders, and hypomania. He divides schizophrenics into subcategories of onion or garlic.

Psychotherapy takes the form of a series of intermittent encounters designed to help a patient accommodate to life's inevitable reoccurring crises and situations. A flexible schedule of sessions is employed and therapists do not keep patients in treatment until every conflict in the recess of the unconscious has been analyzed. The concept of cure is not used in this therapy because it implies that therapy can fix all mental health problems and reinforces the view that all psychological problems are illnesses of which successful therapy can rid the patient.

Once the patient masters the tasks of therapy, he or she leaves treatment and returns only when more help is needed in accommodating to life situations. Once sufficient help is obtained for the presenting problem, this discrete episode of therapy ends. The patient stops seeing the therapist for regular sessions but additional episodes may be expected to recur throughout a patient's life. Termination is not a difficult and painful process, but merely a rapprochement that puts the patient on the path to independence.

Therapy is indicated if and only if the individual needs help learning more effective and adaptive ways of dealing with perceived threats.

Cummings' model constitutes the new broad view of how all therapy ought to be conducted in a modern cultural context. He believes that skilled brief therapy is cost effective as well as therapeutically effective because the patient's problems are brought to rapid resolution.

Intermittent Group Therapy

Although this chapter concentrates on individual therapy, intermittent therapy can be used for groups as well. Based on the same assumptions as intermittent individual therapy, Zimmet (1979; 1989) devised the developmental task and crisis group therapy model, which expands the use of developmental stage theory and crisis intervention to a group therapy format. Persons who are struggling with similar life issues can join together and focus on the psychological work of resolving specific developmental tasks.

The sharing of age- and stage-related issues with similar others reduces feelings of isolation and helps group members negotiate significant transitions throughout their life span.

The Transtheoretical Model of Change

Another model of psychotherapy that can be subsumed under the intermittent therapy model and that possesses the potential to help a varied clinical population is the transtheoretical model of change created and advanced by James O. Prochaska (Prochaska & DiClemente, 1984). This treatment approach integrates effective techniques of the major psychotherapy theories, emphasizes empiricism and outcome measures, accounts for how people change both in and out of therapy, generalizes to changes in health and psychological realms, and is flexible enough to encourage therapists to be creative and innovative. Prochaska highlighted 10 change processes that have received considerable empirical support, including consciousness raising, catharsis, self-reevaluation, environmental reevaluation, self-liberation, social liberation, counterconditioning, stimulus control, contingency management, and the helping relationship. Furthermore, people choose a method of change that depends on where they are in the process. Empirical data support the idea that change occurs in stages.

In Stage 1, *precontemplation,* the individual is unaware or underaware of his or her problems and does not intend to change. This person does little or nothing to overcome his or her problem and is often labeled "resistant" by therapists. Often he or she comes to therapy coerced by an outside force such as a relative, an employer, or the courts. In Stage 2, *contemplation,* the person is aware that a problem is exists but is not committed to taking any action. This individual increases cognitive, affective, and evaluative functioning about the problem and knows what solution is desired or where he or she would like to go, but is not yet ready to go there. In Stage 3, *preparation,* the individual shows a readiness to change and develops an action plan for how he or she will proceed. This person aims to take action and makes small behavioral changes. In Stage

4, *action,* the individual modifies his or her behavior, performs overt behaviors, and invests the necessary time and energy to settle his or her problems. This individual acts from a sense of self-liberation. In Stage 5, *maintenance,* the individual builds on each process to sustain change. This person strives to prevent relapse and to consolidate the gains achieved during action.

To progress in a linear fashion through the stages is the exception. Relapse is the rule. Recycling through the stages in a spiral pattern is common. Difficulties or problems end when the individual is no longer tempted to return to the problem behavior and does not need to expend effort to prevent backsliding. The therapist expects that the patient will return to therapy for booster sessions when the patient feels as though he or she is losing ground.

The transtheoretical model holds that change is an element common to all types of therapies. Each patient is in a particular stage of change when he or she enters therapy. Treatment of all patients as though they are in the same stage of change is ineffectual. A therapist must be able to identify which stage of change a given patient is in when entering therapy in order to assess that patient rapidly and efficiently, to select the best therapeutic methods, and to maximize therapeutic gain. Thus, an effective therapist needs to be an expert on the process of change. It follows logically that the therapist differentially applies different change processes at specific stages of change. For example, the offering of support has a different effect on the patient who is in the precontemplation stage of change than on the patient who is in the maintenance stage. The parameters of therapy vary according to both the stage and the level of change, as well as how much homework clients perform. Thus, the model holds promise to produce stage-matched interventions to maximize therapeutic progress and gains.

There is an increasing body of research on which the stages of change are based. Research actually guides practice, which means that clinicians can choose with confidence which interventions are most effective. Understanding of such universal variables is a way to unite the common elements of psychotherapy and to devise cost-effective care.

When elements of intermittent therapy throughout the life style are combined with the model of transtheoretical change, an efficient view of therapy emerges. The therapist who functions as the psychological family doctor can work with the patient to determine the stage of change and can function as a mental health expert with a realistic point of view who understands how and why people change.

Single Session Therapy

The briefest of the brief therapies is single session therapy (Bloom, 1992, 1997; Hoyt, Talmon, & Rosenbaum, 1990; Talmon, 1990). Proponents of single session therapy do not claim that most psychological problems can be resolved in one session of therapy. Rather, they assert that research clearly demonstrates that approximately 50% of patients unilaterally terminate therapy after a single session. It behooves the therapist to readjust his or her thinking about what a single session may mean in the life of a patient. The therapist should not limit his or her thinking about a patient who comes for a single session. One session does not necessarily mean the person is a "drop out" who was unsuitable for psychotherapy or that the therapist failed due to an inability to retain a therapy candidate. Instead, the therapist ought to see the single session as a unique encounter and a one-time opportunity to help. Because epidemiological data show that so many people come for only a single session, the therapist ought to act as though every session is the only one. The first session makes a lasting impression on the patient and also sets the stage for future therapy. Thus, with the attitude that this meeting may be the one and only mental health intervention that this person receives at this time in life, the therapist should try to make it the most powerful and the best treatment intervention possible. In the single session perspective, the therapist chooses the nature of the focus (i.e., intrapsychic, characterological, interpersonal, or systemic approaches) and then selects appropriate interventions from among educational, behavioral, psychodynamic, systemic, experiential, and medical techniques. Therapists should use succinct, effective, short-term techniques, which include the following: identify the focal problem, formulate comments in 10 words or less, be active, make interpretations tentatively, encourage the expression of affect, keep track of time, keep factual questions to a minimum, do not be overly concerned about the precipitating event, do not overestimate or underestimate the patient's ability, use psychoeducation, mobilize social supports, start a problem-solving process, and build in a follow-up plan.

Interpersonal–Developmental–Existential Therapy

Developed by Budman and Gurman (1988) at the Harvard Health Care Plan, the interpersonal–developmental–existential (I-D-E) model of psychotherapy has the therapist conceptualize the client's problems as "core issues." Client problems are categorized according to several major themes. These include topics of interpersonal and existential losses, developmental lags, specific symptoms and habit disorders, interpersonal complaints, and personality disorders.

In order to arrive at an appropriate I-D-E focus for a particular patient, the therapist obtains information such as why the patient is seeking therapy now, which stage of development the patient is at and what the pertinent life-cycle issues facing him or her are, what, if any, significant anniversaries are taking place, what kinds of social support systems the patient might have, whether any chemical dependency problems are present, whether any outside forces are exerting pressure on the individual to come in for therapy, what the responses to prior treatment have been, and whether the patient wants limited symptom relief or other types of changes. The therapist uses eclectic methods to help the patient reach his or her goals including as psychodynamic, behavioral, and hypnotic interventions; individual, group, marital treatment formats; and between-session homework assignments as needed.

Strategic/Solution-Focused Approach

Ellen Quick's (1996) strategic/solution-focused approach toward therapy is an outgrowth of her experience in managed care settings. It is an interactional, constructivist method that integrates strategic approaches and solution-focused models of psychotherapy. This method appears to be extremely useful in enhancing patient problem solving. It focuses on precise clarification of the patient's problem with emphasis on detailed exploration of the solution.

The theory can be summarized in three principles: First, what is the problem? (If it is not broken do not fix it.) Second, if it works, do more of it and if it does not work, stop doing it. Finally, do something different. The first step is problem clarification, which begins with the therapist asking the patient, "What is the trouble?" followed by attempts to define the highest priority problem and the way in which it is a problem. The therapist finds out how the patient believes therapy can help. The next step is referred to as solution amplification because it highlights the patient's goals and solutions. The therapist asks the patient the so-called miracle questions, "If you were to wake up tomorrow morning and the problem you are here about were solved, what would be different? What would your significant other notice about you? And how would he or she be different?" The therapist helps the patient find exceptions to the problem to determine whether there are pieces to the solution that are already happening. Assessment of these attempted solutions is then made. In the intervention stage of therapy, the therapist validates the chief complaint, compliments the patient for his or her attempts to solve the problem, and suggests homework assignments. Scaling techniques are used to help the patient estimate the severity of the problem and determine whether improvements have been made. Planning for additional services is flexible and open ended, based on need rather than on custom. There is no predetermined number of sessions, and the schedule of appointments is intermittent.

Possibility-Oriented Psychotherapy

Possibility therapy encourages the patient to use his or her own resources to identify and reach a well-specified goal. According to Friedman and Fangor (1991), this model of therapy stresses the adaptation of wellness as a treatment goal, and downplays pathology and formal psychiatric diagnosis. The methods of this model include an emphasis on patient strengths by emphasizing health and wellness and positive expectancy. The following principles guide the therapy: (a) think small, (b) complicated situations do not require complicated solutions, (c) take the client's resources seriously, (d) therapist and patient should collaborate to create a context for change, (e) choose small defined goals, (f) do just one thing differently, (g) the client contains the seeds of the solution, (h) change is inevitable, (i) help to form a supportive network, and (j) maintain an optimistic stance about change. The therapist begins by using the most parsimonious interventions. He or she centers on solutions, maintains focus on the initial request, uses possibility language, stresses resources and strengths, reframes difficulties in developmental contexts, communicates a sense of humor, and maintains an attitude that shows an awareness of the benign absurdity of life.

Pathogenic Belief Model

The pathogenic belief model is a psychodynamically informed model of therapy created by James Donovan (1987) at Harvard Health Care Plan. Donovan maintains that a crippling self belief, which is a long-standing attempt to solve unresolvable conflicts, maintains a negative pattern of interpersonal relationships for individual patients. Although the person used this defense successfully for survival in childhood, such defense manufactures bad feelings in adulthood. The therapist helps the patient to reframe the pathogenic belief and find more productive self-constructions.

The three phases of psychotherapy include searching for the pathogenic belief, reversing the past trauma, and reframing the belief. No judgmental or confrontational events occur during the initial empathy-building process. Reframing of the pathogenic belief, the key to a successful therapy, is accomplished through the therapist offering him or herself as an alternative object, increasing self-awareness on the part of the patient, and supporting the nontraumatic self–object therapist–patient interactions. A successful outcome means the patient is able to suspend unconscious guilt and is freer to conduct the business of his or her life.

Models of Therapy for Specific Populations in Managed Care Setting

Following is a concise introduction to a variety of approaches that utilize nontraditional interventions with difficult clinical populations.

Personality Disorders.   Strosahl (1991) described a group cognitive behavioral treatment model used at Group Health Cooperative. In this model the therapist teaches patients to identify, challenge, and correct distorted beliefs that result in their dysfunctional lifestyles. In the 14-session group therapy, patients can learn to challenge what causes dysfunctional behavior, to make changes in thinking, to develop behavioral skills to increase interpersonal effectiveness and conflict resolution, and finally to prevent relapse and change maintenance skills. Strosahl reported that nearly 80% of patients who used this method achieved at last one therapeutic objective. Thus, concrete, feasible, and practical guidelines were able to help patients achieve their goals.

Adolescents.   Adams (1991) introduced a model of therapy for adolescents and their families in which patients have up to six visits to solve any crisis. The therapy approach mobilizes family members' coping responses, encouraging them to find social supports to sustain any changes they make. Issues dealt with include parenting, stepparenting, attention deficit disorders, separation and divorce, medical/psychosocial chronic illness, enuresis, and encopreses.

The Chronic Patient.   DeStefano and Henault (1991) described creative and flexible methods used at Community Health Care Plan of New Haven, Connecticut, for treatment of chronic mental patients. Their treatment methods include rapid assessment, intermittent therapy, pharmacotherapy, and family and social involvement in treatment. Social support networking is emphasized, as is finding and maintaining meaningful work. Infrequent individual therapy; supportive group therapy; and collaboration among mental health, medical providers, and family and community support systems produce a treatment environment that has kept individuals who have serious psychological problems well integrated in the community. Furthermore, the combination of individual and group therapy for older chronic patients has proven to be successful in keeping patients from being hospitalized (Austad & Henault, 1989).

Depression and Anxiety.   Professionals know that people who suffer from depression and anxiety disorders can be treated with a number of effective short-term models. The effectiveness of Aaron Beck's cognitive therapy of depression and anxiety and Klerman's interpersonal therapy have undeniable empirical support. These models fit well into managed care settings and are useful in combination with pharmacotherapy (Bloom, 1992, 1997; Schulberg & Scott, 1991).

Pediatrics.   At the request of pediatricians in their managed care setting, Hermann and Cofresi (1994) devised a pediatric mental health consultation model to help families who needed mental health care but who were reluctant to pursue services because they feared being stigmatized, were unable to afford copayments, or could not obtain transportation. In this model, mental health consultants meet with the patient, the pediatrician, and other nonmedical providers. A two-session follow-up is conducted. The patient can be referred for mental health treatment, referred to community services, or told that no further intervention is needed. The originators of this project took outcome measures of patient and pediatrician satisfaction, which showed that levels of both were high.

Older Patients.   Robinson (1994) offers a program at Group Health Cooperative of Puget Sound that integrates the medical and behavioral care of older individuals. Outcome data from several group programs have successfully facilitated changes in patients in the areas of medical compliance, networking, decrease of subjective distress level. A group therapy for depressed older women was run at a New Haven staff model HMO. The group, held every other week, served as a source of support for older women confronted with various diseases and family crises.

Use of Intermittent Therapy and the Process of Change

The case of Monique and Dr. Barbera illustrates how a therapist can use intermittent psychotherapy throughout the life cycle and the stages of change to guide, support, and significantly influence a patient throughout her life cycle.

When Dr. Barbera and Monique first met, Monique was an adolescent who was shy, retiring, and easily intimidated. She was afraid of interacting with the therapist and had to be coaxed into the therapy room by her dominating parents. Monique's school performance was poor. She was failing out of school when she made a suicide attempt after a young man had rejected her advances. Monique had mustered up every ounce of her courage to talk to this young man. She was devastated when he told her he was interested in one of her closest friends. During this initial crisis, Dr. Barbera met with Monique several times a week individually and also met with the family several times to help Monique deal with the stress. The family therapy focused upon her parents' overprotectiveness. Within a month, Monique formed a trusting relationship with Dr. Barbera, who moved her from the precontemplation stage to the change stage. At this early age Monique was able to learn new ways to cope with her problems. Dr. Barbera and she used Quick's strategic/solution-focused therapy. Monique was able to see that her shyness was at the root of serious problems and that learning to be assertive would be helpful. She and her therapist developed a treatment plan that included Monique taking acting lessons. Furthermore, her experiences in acting class became grist for the mill in therapy. In a few months, her social interactions became increasingly positive in both quantity and quality.

For 6 weekly individual sessions, Dr. Barbera and Monique used strategic/solution-focused therapy, and Monique learned to use new coping techniques. Monique was receptive to this kind of therapeutic intervention and it seems that her self-image began to improve. Dr. Barbera then referred Monique to a group psychotherapy with other adolescents. Monique attended 20 sessions of group over a year during which time she met with Dr. Barbera any time she wanted to do. She limited her individual meetings with him to 6, as she wanted to rely on the group and fulfill her promise to make Dr. Barbera obsolete as soon as possible. Monique's sense of independence and autonomy were growing, and the emphasis on the group illustrated how important her ability to interacting with peers was at this developmental juncture in her life.

Within a year, Monique's problems had improved sufficiently so that Dr. Barbera and she agreed that they no longer needed to meet in regular sessions. Knowing that she could return anytime she felt the need to do so, Monique met with Dr. Barbera sporadically another 10 times over the next 4 years to grapple with issues of pathogenic beliefs as described by James Donovan.

Six years later, Monique's father died. She returned to Dr. Barbera in order to work through her grief. Within several months of intermittent therapy, she married and had a child of her own. She and her husband subsequently experienced some difficulties agreeing upon child rearing procedures. They consulted with Dr. Barbera, who used cognitive behavior therapy to help the couple to communicate better.

Four years later, Monique experienced major depression. She returned to her psychological family doctor, Dr. Barbera, who intervened with methods from Aaron Beck's cognitive therapy, interpersonal therapy, and pharmacotherapy.

Some 5 years later, when Monique was in her 40s, she again visited her therapist (now 65) and asked for help in mourning her mother's death. Dr. Barbera used Budman and Gurman's model, focusing on the loss. When her individual grief work was done, Monique entered a grief support group, where she gained even greater understanding. Much improved, Monique stopped seeing Dr. Barbera, adding, "I'll call you if I need to; thanks, doc!"

When Monique heard that Dr. Barbera was retiring at the age of 72, she wrote to him to say, "I always long to talk to you about every little problem that arises. But instead, you have taught me well to think not so much about being with you as about what you would say if I were talking with you—how you would help me to identify my own alternatives! Although I haven't been able to see you lately, I have been so busy solving my own problems. I have made you obsolete, so I decided to drop you a letter filling you in on this past few years.

"Now that you are leaving the practice, I want you to know you will never really leave me as long as I am alive, for I carry you in my heart and soul and memory! Thank you for all of the help you have given me over my life."

By envisioning psychotherapy as intermittent throughout the life cycle, Dr. Barbera was free to use any permutation and combination of therapy models, such as those we have discussed, that were most helpful to his patient. He was free to give Monique necessary and sufficient mental health care at crucial developmental points in her life or at times of increased stresses, problems, crisis, or exacerbations of symptoms. And Monique was able to respond to the work by internalizing the guidance of Dr. Barbera. She was successfully able to take necessary therapy on an intermittent basis.

MODELS OF PSYCHOTHERAPY AND FUTURE TRAINING

Because delivery of mental health care services is undergoing serious review, the inevitable result is an increased focus on developing cost-effective psychotherapy. The challenge is to find a way to practice therapy by developing and using models of psychotherapy that work well and fit within managed care settings.

When therapists combine intermittent therapy throughout the life cycle with elements of the transtheoretical models of change, a new therapy paradigm emerges. High-quality long-term care can be rendered, which shows that such treatment does not have to be traditional long-term therapy with the patient meeting weekly or more with the ambitious goal of restructuring the patient's character. Rather, a family practice model, where the role of the therapist is similar to that of the family doctor, can adequately tend to the needs of many individuals in need of mental health consultation. It is possible to envision psychotherapy as a series of intermittent encounters designed to help a patient accommodate to life's inevitable reoccurring crises and situations. Therapy can continue over a long period of time. Seeing therapy from this perspective is a way to increase the likelihood that those who need psychotherapy will receive it.

To train psychotherapists in the future, these elements must be integrated into education. As professionals, we need to place our energy into helping as many individuals as possible by using therapy models that are based on what therapists and patients actually do rather than on some theoretical model that details how the patient ought to behave (Phillips, 1985). Therapists will find it extremely rewarding to practice psychotherapy in a way that helps many people in a short period of time. As we enter the 21st century, during which economics and managed care will inevitably shape psychotherapy, let us work toward making service delivery changes in a humanitarian way. Mental health professionals and trainees must realize that the mental health care system is dysfunctional, in that millions who are uninsured or underinsured can be helped only if we adhere to a social ethic that values universal health care. As professionals, we must find ways to distribute psychotherapy and other health care resources based on need and medical necessity. The newer models of therapy reviewed here offer one such way to accomplish this goal.

REFERENCES

Adams, J. (1991). Family crisis intervention and psychosocial care for children and adolescents. In C. S. Austad & W. H. Berman (Eds.), *Psychotherapy in managed health care: The optimal use of time and resources.* Washington, DC: American Psychological Association Press (pp. 111–126).

Appelbaum, P. S. (1993). Legal liability and managed care. *American Psychologist, 48*(3), 251–257.

Austad, C. S. (1992). Psychotherapists in independent practice and in managed health care settings: A comparison. *Psychotherapy in Private Practice* 1–6.

Austad, C. S. (1993) Health care reform, managed mental health care, and short-term psychotherapy. In L. VandeCreek, S. Knapp, &T. L. Jackson (Eds.), *Innovations in clinical practice* (pp. 241–256). Sarasota, FL: Professionals Resource Press.

Austad, C. S. (1996a). Can psychotherapy be conducted effectively in managed care settings? In A. Lazarus (Ed.), *Controversies in managed mental health care* (pp. 229–249). Washington, DC: American Psychiatric Press.

Austad, C. S. (1996b). *Is long-term psychotherapy unethical? Toward a social ethic in an era of managed care.* San Francisco, Jossey–Bass.

Austad, C., & Berman, W. (1991). HMO psychotherapy. In C. S. Austad & W. H. Berman (Eds.), *Psychotherapy in managed health care: The optimal use of time and resources* (pp. 5–19). Washington, DC: American Psychological Association Press.

Austad, C. S., & Henault, K. (1989). Group psychotherapy with elderly women. *HMO Practice, 3*(2) 70–71.

Austad, C. S., & Hoyt, M. (1992). The managed care movement and the future of psychotherapy. *Psychotherapy, 29*(1), 109–118.

Austad, C. S., Hunter, R., & Morgan, T. (1998). Managed care, ethics, and psychotherapy. *Clinical Psychology,* 67–76.

Austad, C. S. A., Kisch, J., & DeStefano, L. (1989). The health maintenance organization. II. Implications for psychotherapy. *Psychotherapy, 25*(3), 449–454.

Austad, C. S., & Sherman, W. O. (1992). The psychotherapist and managed care: How will practice be affected? *Psychotherapy in Private Practice, 11*(2), 1–9.

Austad, C. S. Sherman, W. O., Morgan, T., & Holstein, L. (1992). The psychotherapist and the managed care setting. *Professional Psychology: Research and Practice 23*(4), 329–332.

Barlow, D. H. (1996). The effectiveness of psychotherapy: Science and policy. *Clinical psychology, 3*(3), 236–240.

Bauer, G. P., & Kobos, J. C. *Brief therapy: Short-term psychodynamic intervention.* Northvale, NJ: Jason Aronson.

Bennett, M. (1984). Brief psychotherapy and adult development. *Psychotherapy, 21,* 171–176, 1984.

Bennett, M. (1988). The greening of the HMO. *American Journal of Psychiatry, 145* (12), 1544–1549.

Benson, H., & Stuart, M. (1992). *The wellness book.* New York: Birch Lane Press.

Bergin, A. E. (1992). Achievements and limitations of psychotherapy research. In D. K. Freedheim (Ed.), *History of psychotherapy.* Washington, DC: American Psychological Association.

Berlin, I. (1969). Resistance to change in mental health professionals. *American Journal of Orthopsychiatry, 39*(1), 109–115.

Bistline, J. L., Sheridan, S. M., & Winegar, M. (1991). Five critical skills for mental health counselors in managed health care. *Journal of Mental Health Counseling, 13*(1), 147–152.

Bloom, B. L. (1990). Managing mental health services: Some comments for the overdue debate in psychology. *Community Mental Health Journal, 26*(1), 107–124.

Bloom, B. (1992). Bloom's focused single session therapy. In Bloom, B. (Ed.), *Planned short term therapy* (pp. 97–121). Boston: Allyn & Bacon.

Bloom, B. (1997). *Planned short-term therapy* (2d ed.). Boston: Allyn & Bacon.

Boaz, J. T. (1988). *Delivering mental health care: A guide for HMOs.* Chicago: Pluribus Press.

Bowers, T., & Knapp, S. (1993). Reimbursement issues for psychologists in independent practice. *Psychotherapy in Private Practice, 12*(3), 73–87.

Budman, S. H., & Gurman, A. S. (1988). *The theory and practice of brief psychotherapy.* New York: Guilford Press.

Callan, M. F., & Yeager, D. C. (1991). *Containing the health care cost spiral.* New York: McGraw–Hill.

Carter, R. (1993, January/February). Mental health policy at a crossroads. *Behavioral Healthcare Tomorrow,* 27–30.

Castro, J. (1994). *The American way of health.* New York: Little, Brown, and Company.

Clemens, N. (1995). Position statement on medical psychotherapy. *American Journal of Psychiatry, 152*(11), 1700.

Cohen, P., & Cohen, J. (1984). The clinician's illusion. *Archives of General Psychiatry, 41,* 1178–1182.

Cummings, N. (1986) The dismantling of our health system. *American Psychologist, 41*(4), 426–431.

Cummings, N. (1991a). Intermittent therapy throughout the life cycle. In C. S. Austad & W. H. Berman (Eds.), *Psychotherapy in managed health care: The optimal use of time and resources* 35–46. Washington, DC: American Psychological Association Press.

Cummings, N. (1991b). The somaticizing patient. In C. S. Austad & W. H. Berman (Eds.), *Psychotherapy in managed health care: The optimal use of time and resources* (pp. 35–46). Washington, DC: American Psychological Association Press.

Cummings, N., Pallak, M., & Cummings, J. (1996). *Surviving the demise of solo practice.* Madison, CT: Psychosocial Press.

Cummings, N., & Sayana, M. (1995). *Focused psychotherapy: A casebook of brief intermittent psychotherapy.* New York: Brunner Mazel.

Dacso, S. T., & Dacso, C. C. (1995). *Managed care answer book.* New York: Aspen.

Davis, G. S. (1990). A managed health care primer. In D. A. Hastings, W. L. Krasner, J. L. Michael, & N. D. Rosenberg (Eds.), *The insiders guide to managed care* (pp. 13–35). Washington, DC: The National Lawyers Association.

Dawes, R. (1994). *House of cards* (pp. 107–120). New York: Free Press.

DeStefano, L., & Henault, K. (1991). The treatment of chronically mentally and emotionally disabled patients. In C. S. Austad & W. H. Berman (Eds.), *Psychotherapy in managed health care: The optimal use of time and resources* (pp. 138–152). Washington, DC: American Psychological Association Press.

Donovan, J. (1987). Brief dynamic psychotherapy: Toward a more comprehensive model. *Psychiatry, 50,* 167–183.

Ellwood, P. (1988, June 9). The Shattuck Lecture—Outcomes management: A technology of patient experience. *New England Journal of Medicine.*

England, M. J., & Cole, R. (1993). Discussion of use of inpatient services by a national population: Do benefits make a difference? *Journal of the American Academy of Child and Adolescent Psychiatry, 32*(1), 153–154.

Feldman, S. (Ed.). (1992). *Managed mental health services.* Springfield, IL: Charles C. Thomas.

Flinn, D. E., McMahon, T. C., & Collings, M. F. (1987). Health maintenance organizations and their implications for psychiatry. *Hospital and Community Psychiatry, 38*(3), 255–263.

Fonagy, P., & Target, M. (1996). Should we allow psychotherapy research to determine clinical practice? *Clinical Psychology, 3*(3), 245–150.

Friedman, S., & Fangor, M. T. (1991). *Expanding therapeutic possibilities: Getting results in brief therapy.* Lexington, MA: Lexington Books.

Garfield, S., & Bergin, A. (1986). Introduction and historical overview. In. S. Garfield & A. Bergen (Eds.), *Handbook of psychotherapy and behavior change* (pp. 3–22). New York: Wiley.

Goran, M. J. (1992). Managed mental health and group insurance. In S. Feldman (Ed.). *Managed mental health services* (pp. 27–43). Springfield, IL: Charles C. Thomas.

Hermann, B., & Cofresi, A. (1994, January). *The pediatric population.* Paper presented at Group Health Institute of America, Miami Beach, FL.

Howard, K. I., Davidson, C., Mahoney, M. T., Orlinsky, D., & Brown, K. P. (1989). Patterns of psychotherapy utilization. *American Journal of Psychiatry, 146*(6), 775–778.

Hoyt, M. F. (1985). Therapist resistances to short-term dynamic psychotherapy. *Journal of the American Academy of Psychoanalysis, 13,* 93–112.

Hoyt, M., & Austad, C. S. (1992). The managed care movement and the future of psychotherapy. *Psychotherapy, 29*(1), 109–118.

Hoyt, M. F., Talmon, M., & Rosenbaum, R. (1990). Planned single session psychotherapy: An analysis of patients self reports. In S. Budman, M. F. Hoyt, & S. Friedman (Eds.), *Casebook of brief psychotherapies.* New York: Guilford Press.

Kleinke, C. (1994). *Common principles of psychotherapy.* Pacific Grove, CA: Brooks/Cole.

Kohrman, C. H. (1986). Medical practice where HMOs dominate: The perspective of physicians in Minneapolis–St. Paul. *Journal of Medical Practice Management, 2*(2), 81–89.

Koss, M. P., & Butcher, J. N. (1986). Research on brief psychotherapy. In S. Garfield & A. Bergin (Eds.), *Handbook of psychotherapy and behavior change* (pp. 627–670). New York: Wiley.

Lambart, M. (1991). Introduction to psychotherapy research. In L. Beutler & M. Crago (Eds.), *Psychotherapy research* (pp. 1–11). Washington, DC: American Psychological Association.

Lambert, M., Shapiro, D., & Bergin, A. (1986). The effectiveness of psychotherapy. In S. Garfield & A. Bergin (Eds.), *The handbook of psychotherapy and behavior change.* New York: Wiley.

Levin, B. L. (1992). Mental health services within the HMO group. *HMO Practice, 6*(3), 16–20.

Newman, F., & Tejeda, M. (1996). The need for research that is designed to support decisions in the delivery of mental health services. *American psychologist, 51*(10), 1040–1049.

Olfson, M., & Pincus, H. (1994). Outpatient psychotherapy in the United States. Part I. Costs, and user characteristics. *American Journal of Psychiatry, 151,* 1281–1288.

Olsen, D. P. (1995). Ethical cautions in the use of outcomes for resource allocation in the managed care environment of mental health. *Archives of Psychiatric Nursing, 9*(4), 173–178.

Phillips, L. (1985). *A guide for therapists and patients to short-term psychotherapy.* Springfield, IL: Charles C. Thomas.

Prochaska, J. O., & DiClemente, C. C. (1984). The transtheoretical approach: Crossing the traditional boundaries of therapy. Homewood, IL: Dow–Jones–Irwin.

Quick, E. K. (1996). *Doing what works in brief therapy.* New York: Academic Press.

Robinson, P. (1994, January). *The elderly.* Paper presented at Group Health Institute of America, Miami Beach, FL.

Rodriguez, A. R. (1994). Quality-of-care guidelines. In R. K. Schreter, S. S. Sharfstein, & C. A. Schreter (Eds.), *Allies and adversaries: The impact of managed care on mental health services* (pp. 169–185). Washington, DC: American Psychiatric Press.

Sabin, J. E. (1994a). Caring about patients and caring about money: The American Psychiatric Association code of ethics meets managed care. *Behavioral Sciences & the Law, 12*(4), 317–330.

Sabin, J. E. (1994b). Ethical issues under managed care. In R. K. Schreter, S. S. Sharfstein, & C. A. Schreter (Eds.), *Allies and adversaries: The impact of managed care on mental health services* (pp. 187–200). Washington, DC: American Psychiatric Press.

Schulberg, H., & Scott, C. P. (1991). Depression in primary care: Treating depression with interpersonal psychotherapy. In C. S. Austad & W. H. Berman (Eds.), *Psychotherapy in managed health care: The optimal use of time and resources* (pp. 153–171). Washington, DC: American Psychological Association Press.

Seligman, M. (1995). The effectiveness of psychotherapy: The Consumer Reports Study. *American Psychologist 50*(12), 969.

Spencer, C. S., IFrank, R. G., & McGuire, T. (1996). How should the profit motive be used in managed care? In A. Lazarus (Eds.), *Controversies in managed mental health care* (pp. 279–290). Washington, DC: American Psychiatric Press.

Starr, P. (1982). *The social transformation of American medicine.* New York: Basic Books.

Stein, L. I. (1994). *Maturing mental health systems: New challenges and opportunities. New directions for mental health services.* San Francisco: Jossey–Bass.

Strosahl, K. (1991). Cognitive and behavioral treatment of the personality disordered patient. In C. S. Austad & W. H. Berman (Eds.), *Psychotherapy in managed health care: The optimal use of time and resources* (pp. 185–202). Washington, DC: American Psychological Association Press.

Talmon, M. (1990). *Single session therapy.* San Francisco, Jossey–Bass.

VandenBos, G. (1986). Psychotherapy research: A special issue [Special issue]. *American Psychologist, 41*(2), 11–112.

Webb, W., Rothschild, B. S., & Monroe, L. (1994). Ethical codes of conduct in the medical profession. In R. E. Hales, S. C. Yudofsky, & J. A. Talbott (Eds.), *Ethics and psychiatry* (pp. 1341–1354). Washington, DC: American Psychiatric Press.

Wilson, (1996). Empirically validated treatments: Reality and resistance. *Clinical Psychology, 3*(3), 241–244.

Zimet, C. (1974). Developmental task and crisis groups: The application of group psychotherapy to maturational processes. *Psychotherapy, Research, and Practice, 16,* 2–8.

Zimet, C. N. (1989). The mental health care revolution: Will psychology survive? *American Psychologist 44*(4), 703–708.

4

Group Psychotherapies and Managed Care

K. Roy MacKenzie
University of British Columbia, Vancouver

This chapter places the use of psychotherapy groups in their historical and conceptual contexts. In particular, it emphasizes the need to examine a number of established clinical traditions that have prevented more extensive use of the group as a treatment modality. These factors are particularly pertinent to the managed care environment in its present imperfect state of development.

HISTORICAL USE OF GROUP THERAPY

Use of group psychotherapy can be traced over several waves of utilization (MacKenzie, 1997b). The first significant use of groups in service systems occurred during the Second World War. The necessity of treating many casualties with psychological distress and limited treatment resources provided an ideal opportunity to introduce group methods. Carl Menninger spoke of group psychotherapy as one of the major treatment advances of the war. However the use of groups in civilian populations did not spread widely until the general social movement toward group activities characteristic of the 1960s and 1970s. The treatment community echoed this trend and there was a proliferation of group methods. This was augmented by passage of the Community Mental Health Centers Act of 1963, which resulted in a surge of interest in developing service programs for a defined clinical population. Despite an enthusiastic beginning, many community mental health centers (CMHC) became focused on the acute treatment of less severely impaired clients and the CMHC movement lost much of its momentum. In the 1980s, a proliferation of effective medications and more sophisticated research technologies led academic psychiatry toward biological mechanisms and a general disregard of psychotherapeutic modalities. Group methods again experienced a decline in support.

65

The managed care industry has shown considerable interest in the use of groups. However, as is discussed in what follows, efforts to implement this goal generally, with some notable exceptions, have not generally been successful. Nonetheless, the current focus on the development of organized service systems for a defined population base provides an opportunity for a resurgence in the use of group psychotherapy models. To achieve this opportunity it is necessary to address potential resistance both in the attitudes of clinicians and the organization of service systems. The present health care context contains many of the same pressures that existed during both the wartime and the CMHC periods of group enthusiasm. For economic reasons, there are again strong pressures to treat a given clinical population in the most cost-effective manner. These pressures in part reflect the rapid rise in health care costs that occurred during the 1980s and into the 1990s before coming under moderate control by 1993.

This chapter is written with the underlying assumption that there will be continuing pressure to manage health care costs and that the majority of clinicians will be connected in some manner to larger systems that influence the flow of referrals (MacKenzie, 1995). This will lead to the further development of service systems that stream patients into the most cost-effective services. These pressures will be counterbalanced by increasing consumer and corporate pressures for quality care. At present this tension is being addressed by legislative and legal challenges that by and large are clumsy efforts to control an extremely complex industry. It remains to be seen how these developments will evolve, though there is a general expectation that larger integrated systems of health care are likely to emerge.

Historically, and still today, the field of group psychotherapy has been a divided and polarized one. The majority of senior group therapists have been trained in psychodynamic models. Groups conducted by these practitioners have generally been structured to provide longer term therapy measured in years. They are typically open groups with a slow turnover of members as group positions become available. Most of the formal group psychotherapy literature is concerned with this type of group model. This is not a model favored by cost-conscious managers.

Another large group of therapists come from public service or managed care programs where emphasis is on psychoeducational and skill-focused groups, often of brief duration. Although it is clearly helpful for some clients, this approach is not designed to address more substantial levels of psychopathology. Such programs may run in parallel with long-term groups that provide a supportive function for chronic populations with major mental illness. The goal for these groups is maintenance and prevention of recurrence more than active change.

Historically, substance abuse programs have also been provided through the group modality, though their roots are in self-help models that have not emphasized traditional therapist-led group psychotherapy methods.

The individual psychotherapy literature has been characterized by a consistent interest in intensive, focused, time-limited models for over two decades (Barber & Crits-Christoph, 1995; MacKenzie, 1996b). The group literature has lagged in this regard but has been gaining strength over the past decade (Mac-Kenzie, 1994a; Steenbarger & Budman, 1996). Many of these models are designed for treatment of a specific diagnostic population. For example, cognitive therapy models have been utilized particularly for depression and several anxiety syndromes (Beck, Rush, Shaw, et al., 1979). Interpersonal models have evolved for acute reactive states that often involve relationship stress, self-esteem, and related depression (Klerman, Weissman, Rounsaville, et al., 1984). The title of this chapter refers to "group psychotherapies" because of the increasing use of group models that are specifically designed for particular diagnostic or other homogeneous client populations. These vary considerably in format, thus making the term "group psychotherapy" itself relatively uninformative.

THE PSYCHOTHERAPY UTILIZATION CURVE

There is a well-established literature concerning the way in which clients use psychotherapy services. Much of this information dates to before the major changes in health care delivery of the past decade. Empirical studies have been quite consistent in their findings. Figure 4.1 reflects several perspectives on psychotherapy utilization.

The dose–response curve of the upper line in Fig. 4.1 is based on statistically significant improvement (Howard, Kopta, Krause, et al., 1986). It is evident that most clients respond quickly to formal therapy, with over 50% improvement within the first 2 months. The rate of response continues to rise, though at

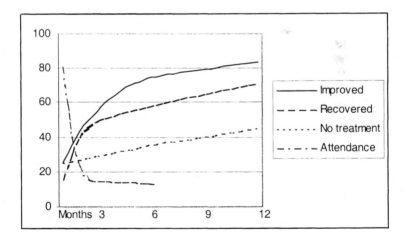

FIG. 4.1.   Composite graph of time progressions: Improved (Howard et al., 1986); Recovered – Chronic Distress Symptoms (Kopta et al., 1994); No treatment (Eysenck, 1952); Attendance (Phillips, 1987).

a somewhat slower rate, over the next 4 months so that by the 6-month point there is a 75% response rate. By the end of 2 years the improvement curve has risen slowly to 85%. This curve reflects an impressive response to psychotherapy, better than many medical treatments.

The second dose–response curve in Fig. 4.1 is based on more recent analyses identifying clinical recovery in terms of more stringent criteria that require symptom measures to have returned to within a statistically normal range (Kopta, Howard, Lowry, & Beutler, 1994; Kadera, Lambert, & Andrews, 1996). This curve rises more slowly but still reaches the improvement curve by about the 6-month point.

For reference purposes, the third change curve reflects the improvement over time of a nontreated clinical population. This curve begins to approach the treated population near the 2-year point. Interestingly, the figures for this particular untreated curve are taken from Eysenck's (1952) article that created a storm of controversy with its assertion that no-treatment patients recovered as much as those who received formal therapy. This curve is consistent with other, more current sources that track the course of untreated nonpsychotic illness. Eysenck's position was correct only if a time frame of 2 years was applied, but in clinical terms, his own data indicate a major positive effect of psychotherapy and a substantial relief of morbidity and dysfunction.

Finally, the bottom curve in Fig. 4.1 suggests that in practice most patients attend relatively few sessions (Phillips, 1987). By the end of 2 months, almost all service systems indicate that only about 20% of those who enter will still remain in active treatment. Once this remaining cohort has reached the 6-month point, it is likely that attendance will continue for a longer period. It is worth noting that this curve is based on data collected prior to the major impact of managed care systems.

These curves constitute a composite picture of change representing many different conditions and depths of dysfunction. Obviously, acute situations related to clear immediate external stress tend to respond quite quickly, whereas long-standing anxiety and depression syndromes respond more slowly, as do severe personality disorders. This perspective on the predictable rates of change of a larger clinical population is a valuable guide in the development of clinical service programs (Vessey, Howard, Lueger, Kachele, & Mergenthaler, 1994) and is used later in this chapter as a template for the development of group programs. However, the curves of Fig. 4.1 make no distinction between the modalities of service delivery; these include individual, group and family treatment approaches, and many different models of psychotherapy.

INDIVIDUAL VERSUS GROUP TREATMENT EFFECTIVENESS

There is a common clinical myth that the group format is satisfactory for providing general support but that individual psychotherapy is required for more effective active treatment. Fortunately there is a substantial empirical literature that addresses this hypothesis (Fuhriman & Burlingame, 1994; Lambert &

Bergin, 1994). Tillitski (1990) reports on 50 studies in which a given type of treatment was provided in an individual or group format. The results are impressively clear: overall there is no difference in outcome. A small number of these studies found individual better, and about the same number found group more effective. Piper and Joyce (1996) and McRoberts, Burlingame, and Hoag (1998) conducted a more stringent review of the literature, restricting the studies to those with sound methodological features and well-defined psychotherapy models. These reviews also found no appreciable difference in outcome.

How, then, can one account for the clear preference in the larger clinician community for individual psychotherapy? Three major issues are commonly found.

The first common reaction is to lay blame at the feet of clients: "Almost everyone I see does not like the idea of group." However, clinical programs that have well-developed group programs report little resistance of this nature.

Certainly training plays a role. Most clinicians have received modest formal supervised training in leading clinical groups. Often this is primarily composed of a smattering of theory and personal experience as the member of a brief group run on group dynamics or psychoanalytic principles. Both of these traditions have value, but for an introductory experience they are often perceived as quite aversive and of course are not directly applicable to a group composed of clients with significant psychological disturbance. These traditions are often accompanied by the inference that real groups are best conceptualized as long term in nature and that briefer models are little more than window dressing for ineffective therapy. It is common to find inexperienced clinicians thrown into groups of clients with significant psychopathology. The predictable result is, at the least, general dissatisfaction or, at the worst, group dissolution or negative clinical effects from scapegoating.

Finally, few service programs have developed effective mechanisms for streaming appropriate clients into suitable groups. This often results in difficulty finding enough members to start groups. Therefore, the groups begin with three or four members and never build up enough steam to provide a satisfying group experience. The leader attempts to combat the small size by focusing on individual members in turn, and the result is diluted and unsatisfying individual therapy. Other groups may be created with membership mixes that work against group cohesion. Often, managed care regulations make no allowance for the expanded scope of coverage in groups and enforce unrealistic restrictions on the number of sessions, making the development of a working group atmosphere near impossible. Others insist on immediate admission to treatment so that there is little opportunity to compose a group that is likely to be successful.

The litany of difficulties just discussed commonly reflect a failure to make the transition from conceptualizing the application of group psychotherapy as a single long-term group to viewing it as a set of many groups that are part of a service delivery system. The remainder of this chapter focuses on aspects of developing groups in a variety of time frames and for a range of purposes as well as the development of structured service systems. If the prediction earlier in this chapter that most psychotherapy services will be conducted within the framework of a larger service system is correct, then the use of groups should have a positive future. The larger flow of potential group members that a service system can provide is an ideal context for the use of groups. The realization of this goal is dependent on a flexible attitude about the nature of clinical groups and the creation of a superstructure that can facilitate introduction of the right client into the right group in the right time frame.

TRADITIONAL MODEL OF GROUP PROCESS

In a later section, specific models of group psychotherapy for specific purposes are discussed. However, the group literature runs in parallel with the individual literature in identifying a number of common factors that underlie effective group work of all kinds (Winston & Muran, 1996).

Groups provide a more complex and multifaceted field for interaction than does individual therapy (Bernard & MacKenzie, 1994). This brings with it a dilution of the power hierarchy. In individual therapy the therapist and the client remain in a clear control imbalance no matter how egalitarian the therapist attempts to be. In groups, most of the therapeutic action stems from interactions among members. The therapist is a step removed, striving to achieve a constructive group environment through which such therapeutic intermember action can occur.

It is essential that the clinician making the transition from individual to group work understand the idea of the group system. A helpful way to conceptualize this is to think of several levels of organization to the group. The first is the level of the entire group: "The group feels very close" or "It sounds as if there is a lot of dissatisfaction in the air today." Then it is useful to identify subgroups that may distract from the group work or that may provide opportunities for important clarification work concerning their different perspectives: "Perhaps those of you on each side of this issue could explore your differences more directly." Within a given group, there are numerous opportunities to focus on the interactions between two specific members: "A lot of tension seems to be generated between the two of you; can you say some more about what it's about?" Finally, each member has internal issues to deal with: "It appears that you are struggling with whether to be in the group or separate from it." The leader has the option of which level to choose for interventions. In general, the most important task is to use the interactional levels to encourage group level learning and application.

A group in which the members are actively interacting with one another will progress rapidly in the direction of greater group cohesion. This notion of the group "esprit de corp" is parallel to the "alliance" in the individual literature (MacKenzie, 1998). A group that lacks cohesion is much weaker in its capacity to influence positive change in the individual members.

The group literature has emphasized the role of group therapeutic factors. A subset of four supportive factors are particularly important in the early stages of the group. (a) *Universality* refers to the experiencing of common issues among the members. This process begins almost with the first words spoken in a group: "That sounds just like what I've been experiencing." Universality may be built on relatively superficial issues in the beginning, but the important aspect is that it brings the group members closer and enhances a sense of safety. (b) *Acceptance* by the group is a more complex and powerful experience than that normally found in individual therapy. It provides a solid base for enhancement of self-esteem. (c) *Altruism* provides the individual member with the opportunity to be of value to others, which is also a strong mechanism for self-worth. (d) These three interactional mechanisms create a climate in which hope that change is possible can develop.

It is obvious that cohesion and the supportive factors will reinforce one another. The primary task of the leader in a newly formed group is to enable the members to actively interact with one another so that these mechanisms can operate effectively. It should be noted that all of these factors with the exception of hope are unique to the group environment. Proper attention to these aspects of groupness ensures that the group can move on to deeper work. The promotion of the supportive factors is technically simple. The leader can provide firm support for members actively talking to one another, and not to the leader. The supportive factors will emerge automatically and the therapist may need to be careful not to get in the way. They can be subtlety reinforced by comments such as, "What was it like finding that the two of you have had similar experiences?" "Maybe we could end this first session by reviewing how comfortable members are in the group," "It sounded like your comment was helpful to her."

A final aspect of the generic group is that of group development. This has been clearly identified in empirical process research (MacKenzie, 1994a, 1997a). A simple schema for group development consists of four stages: engagement, differentiation, interpersonal work, and termination. The engagement stage depends heavily on the cultivation of cohesion and the supportive factors. It ends when all members appear connected to the group and are participating to at least a modest extent. This stage is based on recognition of similarities. The differentiation stage leads to a more confrontational atmosphere where differences are explored. This stage also raises the challenge of dealing with negative affect. Once these two stages have been mastered, usually within the first six sessions of a weekly outpatient group, the group is in a position to conduct more active interpersonal learning. The termination of an active group brings with it echoes of existential issues (MacKenzie, 1996a). These include dealing with issues of loss and grief, of not getting as much as one would like, and of taking responsibility for oneself. These phenomena of group development and termination are particularly powerful when the entire group starts and ends together.

This material concerning the common features of the group has been emphasized because these phenomena occur in all groups, including those in which group process is not planned to be a central focus. The leader must track these group system characteristics to ensure that they are developing as anticipated or at least being managed effectively. For example, a group that lacks cohesion is not simply failing to progress. It may be exerting a powerful negative effect that decreases motivation and effective application of the material to be learned. A group with unresolved tension between some of the members may become actively destructive through scapegoating pressures.

These warnings are particularly relevant for clinicians working in managed care systems. Many such systems have administrative rules in place that actively mitigate against effective group therapy. This is a paradox because it is not uncommon for the same systems to express a strong interest in increasing the use of groups. Usually any difficulties are the result of ignorance more than intent. Some of the more common problems are addressed in the next section.

GROUP PSYCHOTHERAPY PROGRAMS
IN MANAGED CARE SETTINGS

It is important that the clinician think in terms of group programs, not simply doing some groups (MacKenzie, 1997b; Crosby & Sabin, 1996). The principal cause of difficulty in expanding the use of groups resides in a failure to consider service delivery issues. The first portion of this section considers a range of group models. This material is then applied to groups in formal integrated systems. The final section applies these ideas to solo practitioners or smaller consortiums of arm's length practitioners. For all of these contexts, the clinician needs to consider the appropriate range of group models. This list of implementation challenges is not intended to discourage the use of groups, but rather to highlight issues that will emerge in most programs. To be forewarned is to be forearmed.

Applying the Time Categories of the Dose-Response Curve

(1) The first segment of the dose–response curve (Fig. 4.1) deals with therapy of up to about eight sessions

For the front line general mental health service this time frame is likely to accommodate about 50% of those being assessed. The brief time and the high turnover rate make this category less than ideal for the use of groups. However, several specific models have been developed for this purpose using crisis intervention theory. For example, a rapid access group may meet weekly, or more often, with an expected change in membership every session. The sessions are highly structured with a series of go-arounds so individual members are the primary focus, with the group offering feedback, ideas, and encouragement. Practical goals set for each member to work on between sessions are set. A limit is set for maximum attendance, probably not more than eight sessions, and it may not be necessary for a client to attend sequential sessions but to extend the duration of attendance over 3 or 4 months. Such groups are designed for supportive work to address a current issue, not for exploratory psychotherapy. The leaders need to keep this in mind even though the group may become surprisingly evocative at times.

This type of group has much in common with inpatient ward groups. Referral criteria need to specify that the group is not able to contain serious potential for self or other physical harm. Experienced cotherapists are indicated, at least one of whom should be quite knowledgeable about community resources. This is not a group for neophyte leaders.

(2) The next segment of the utilization curve extends from about 12 to 26 sessions

This is the range that has been applied in most of the literature on time-limited therapies. More ambitious intensive therapy goals can be addressed. All time-limited models emphasize the importance of establishing specific goals. An active therapist stance is required to keep to the focus and still maintain a strong working alliance. This requires a careful assessment process to develop a collaborative agreement about focus as well as to prepare and motivate the client for therapeutic work. Two principal methods are generally applied.

Groups Based on Specific Diagnostic Criteria. The most common application of this employs the use of formal DSM-IV diagnostic categories. This is particularly appropriate when a specific therapy model has been designed for the diagnosis. For example, both cognitive-behavior therapy (CBT) and interpersonal psychotherapy (IPT) were created to treat major depression. Several of the anxiety subcategories, such as panic, phobia, and obsessive–compulsive disorder, have unique therapeutic techniques composed of different combinations of behavioral and cognitive strategies. Bulimia nervosa is commonly treated in groups, often with a combination of cognitive and interpersonal focus. Intensive personal therapeutic work with applied application to outside circumstances is anticipated in these groups. Most of these models are relatively complex, and specific training in both the model and its application in a group format is required for their successful application.

General Interpersonal Groups. These groups share many of the techniques of the previously mentioned groups, but place more emphasis on learning from the group interaction. This approach is particularly helpful for issues of self-esteem and entrenched dysfunctional interpersonal patterns. Various methods of establishing a more complex focus, designed to identify dysfunctional relationship patterns and self-perpetuating relationship cycles, are available. Although these assessment procedures are based on an understanding of earlier childhood experiences, the application of them is maintained primarily in current situations. These groups offer more possibilities of process complications and require leaders who are experienced in such techniques.

Situational Groups. Groups may also be formed, not so much by diagnosis, as by situation. Examples of these would be grief groups, divorce/separation groups, and preretirement groups. These groups vary in their balance between group process and leader-centered informational content (McKay & Paleg, 1992). The therapist needs to be clear about what model is being used.

Psychoeducational/Skills Group. A range of groups dealing with specific topic areas in an educational/skill development format may be considered. The range of possibilities is large, including eating disorder psychoeducational groups, stress management groups, assertiveness training groups, family communication groups, and childhood development groups. These formats make less use of the group process and tend to be leader centered. Nonetheless, the group format provides general properties of the supportive therapeutic factors that reinforce motivation and amplify learning. Leaders require less intensive training in group therapy, but must be alert to group management problems. Ready access to clinical supervision is advised.

This emphasis on specific models has a sound rationale. The use of a group format and the imposition of a time limit combine to pose limitations on what can be accomplished. Specific models provide clear guidelines to follow that are generally outlined in clinical manuals. These serve to keep the therapist on track, and outcome research indicates that the following of such guidelines results in more predictable positive outcomes. Most manuals, particularly for diagnosis-specific groups, primarily deal with positioning strategies for the therapist, leaving reasonable room for clinical flexibility. Psychoeducational and situational groups increasingly move into a classroom atmosphere that provides greater emphasis on the learning of designated material. It is likely that clinicians will be expected to justify their choice of model in light of the empirical knowledge, as well as their competence to provide such a model.

Development of Groups in Integrated Service Systems

Although the exact nature of the future mental health service system is unclear, it seems likely that the process of integration of service delivery will continue. Most clinicians are likely to find themselves interacting with these systems in some manner. Larger systems offer some clear advantages for the development of group programs. The larger flow of clients coming through a common assessment stream provides the opportunity to offer a diverse range of groups and to stream clients into the most appropriate group. This sensible goal has proven difficult to achieve in many systems.

Rather than trying to lay out an ideal model which could never fit every setting, the following discussion is centered around a series of issues that commonly present hurdles that must be overcome. Managed care systems have been coming under pressure from clients, legislators, and the courts to ensure that adequate services are provided. This has provided an opening for clinicians to take a proactive stance with regard to the design of treatment services. The challenge for clinicians is to accept that there are funding limitations and that service effectiveness will be monitored. In terms of group programming, it may be helpful to realize that all systems have to struggle with similar challenges and that these are systems issues and not necessarily the result of management personality aberrations. Clinicians with group expertise may make an important contribution to developing a group program. In the process, of course, they are carving out an important role for themselves.

BARRIERS TO GROUP PROGRAMMING AND STRATEGIES FOR DEVELOPING A GROUP PROGRAM

There are many institutional and attitudinal barriers that may hinder the development of groups. Some of them are identified in what follows, along with suggestions for facilitating change.

Attitudinal Issues

(1) Lack of Senior Administrative Support for the Use of Groups

Trying to get groups going without higher sanctions can be a frustrating experience. Institutional bias against the use of groups is rampant, often reflected in inadequate space or time allowance. Referrals keep getting lost, if they come at all, and no one seems to care. The solution is a serious discussion, maybe accompanied by a formal proposal, with senior management. Most systems are beginning to understand that there are advantages to the use of groups but they don't how to proceed. A sensible plan that takes into account the constraints that management might be facing and that outlines the service advantages may lead to a breakthrough. Documentation from the literature is always helpful.

(2) Senior Administration Wants All Therapy to Be Conducted in Groups

Programs that mandate all clients into groups generally come to regret the decision. Client complaints begin to pile up and clinician dissatisfaction rises as inappropriate referrals accumulate. These are the sorts of signs that accreditation bodies can easily identify. As previously noted, a sensible plan that acknowledges the concerns of management may be helpful. This might include criteria that clearly identify inappropriate clients.

(3) Empirical Models But No Empirical Guidelines

Much emphasis has been placed on the use of empirically validated treatment models for both individual and group psychotherapy. Overall this emphasis is likely to have a positive effect, particularly in shrinking the vast array of approaches that may be taken for the same condition. But the devil is in the details, so to speak. Often suitability criteria are ignored, time limits are unrealistically brief, or in some way an essential aspect of the treatment is blocked. This problem may reflect administrative decisions that are based on general principles without a true clinical appreciation of the implications. It is useful to keep in mind that there is also a long-standing tradition of longer term therapy for conditions that are likely to respond to time-limited approaches. The solution to this problem resides in clear and agreed on criteria for referral decisions. This is addressed in more detail later.

(4) Limits on the Number of Sessions

This widespread concern is likely to exist for some time. The dose–response curve is of some help in addressing the question of time. Some systems have taken the fact that most clients do not use more than a handful of sessions and translated it into a policy statement. As in the preceding item, this issue is focused on openly acknowledged assessment criteria.

The zone that is in danger of being underutilized is that of the formal time-limited models lasting for several months. This time category is appropriate for persistent problems that have not responded to brief intervention of six or eight sessions, and group formats are well adapted to these problems. Intensive work requires well-trained and experienced clinicians who are familiar with highly focused techniques. It should be anticipated that a given client might use this format at intervals, particularly at times of specific stress.

The most critical time decision lies at about the 6-month point. Clients who move beyond this enter a chronic care phase of treatment where active change is slower. Difficult diagnostic groups may require special management or programming. For instance, severe personality problems may require 1 to 2 years for significant change to occur and more traditional therapy is generally required. However, it is realistic to expect some cost-offset benefits in terms of reduced days in hospital and emergency room visits. Another area that requires special consideration is long-term management of chronic illness, such as bipolar disorder, chronic depression, and schizophrenia. Services for such patients may often rely on less intensive programming through monthly sessions. Groups offer a suitable format for this purpose.

Outcome studies and cost-offset data indicate that alternative treatment models are worthwhile over a longer time perspective (Gabbard, Lazar, Hornberger, & Spiegel, 1997). If, as seems likely, health care systems become more stabilized, there is reason to expect that the short-term bottom line approach will yield to a longer term perspective of managing a defined population over years so that effective treatment will pay off over time.

This elaboration on time categories of treatment is provided to supply further preparation for addressing issues of severe time restriction in service systems. A clinical proactive stance in defining criteria for purpose-built groups that are designed to maximize use of clinical resources is one way to provide leadership in program design.

(5) Substituting Group for Individual Sessions

In a survey conducted by the National Registry of Certified Group Psychotherapists (1996), it was found that a large majority of managed care companies do not have a code for group sessions: A visit is a visit. This makes little economic sense and clearly prejudices against the use of groups. One of the major attractions of groups in managed systems is the potential for greater cost efficiency. It can be argued that providing an option of three group sessions for one individual session is realistic. This assumes that groups are maintained at a reasonable size, in the 6 to 10 member range for intensive groups, and perhaps somewhat larger for psychoeducational and skill-focused groups. This simple accounting shift would provide a major incentive to develop a larger group program as well as provide clinicians with a more satisfying opportunity to adequately treat more challenging patients with somewhat longer duration of therapy.

(6) Expectation of Immediate Access to Treatment

Many programs have guidelines concerning how quickly a client is engaged in treatment. In a general sense this makes for good policy and better client satisfaction. However, as is discussed in what follows, closed groups that cannot be opened at random to accommodate a new referral offer several advantages. Most clients can appreciate this dilemma and are willing to await the opening of a new group, "their group," if a clear time is established for this. Making accommodation for this possibility greatly assists in the development of an effective group program.

(7) Group Program Coordinator

It is unrealistic to expect a group program to flourish without a clinician being identified as the coordinator with time assigned for the task. In moderate-sized programs this usually requires half time and in larger programs closer to full time. The coordinator is responsible for a number of functions: planning a suitable spectrum of groups, maintaining an effective referral system, promoting groups within the system, probably providing clinical supervision, and generally troubleshooting the service.

Clinician-Driven Barriers

(1) Compensation for Extended Responsibility

Leading a group brings with it a significant extension of clinical responsibility. In return for this, coupled with the increased per-hour benefits to the system, there needs to be some tangible acknowledgment to the clinician. This may come in the form of direct financial benefit, higher service points, lower intake assessment expectations, or access to benefits such as courses and conferences. Some systems have found their group programs faltering and on examination determined that there was a direct penalty for doing groups. If clinicians refer clients to a group, those clinicians lose those clients from their registered caseload. Altering this response lost system results in a major improvement in group referrals.

(2) Time for Record Maintenance

Group therapy requires significantly more time for charting and conducting other administrative functions proportional to time spent with an individual client. This needs to be built into the time schedule. In general, a 2-hour time allowance for a 90-minute group is adequate.

(3) Training and Supervision

Training in individual psychotherapy does not automatically confer expertise in group psychotherapy. In fact, clinicians who are highly experienced in individual work may find it particularly difficult to adapt to a conceptualization of the whole group and to focus on group interaction more than individual internal issues. It may be worthwhile in a larger program desiring to promote more group work to develop a series of in-service training programs. Some type of clinical, not administrative, supervision needs to be built into a group program. The pull of the group environment has the capacity to shift therapists off base. This applies to clinicians running more structured groups as well as those in more intensive formats. The services of the group coordinator may be of value in this regard. At the very least, a regularly scheduled meeting of all therapists conducting groups can be helpful. The opportunity to compare formats, discuss critical incidents, and generally reflect on one's work is helpful in avoiding the development of problematic situations.

(4) Use of Cotherapy

There are few types of groups in which cotherapy is essential, although there are some in which is desirable, for example, in adolescent groups, in couples groups, and as a training format. It is important to understand that cotherapy is a more complex and challenging format with opportunity for undesirable control issues between therapists and for splitting efforts by group members. Above all, the use of cotherapy because of apprehension about running a group alone is the worst rationale for choosing such therapy unless it is part of a planned training exercise. Because cotherapy virtually doubles the staff costs of doing group work, it is not likely to thrive in many service systems.

Organizational Barriers

(1) Serving the Needs of a Population

Health care systems turn the usual incentives around; rather than trying to find enough patients to begin a group, the challenge is to find enough clinicians to manage the required services. Unless there has been a major change in the structure of the system and its potential clients, utilization patterns stay roughly the same from year to year. A good way to begin planning for groups is to review utilization patterns for the preceding year. This might include the distribution of sessions to see if it approximates the dose–response curve. A breakdown into major diagnostic categories is informative. The percentage of clients who received their therapy in a group format is also useful. With this information, a plan for the coming year should be possible.

There is a major advantage to thinking in terms of an annual plan. Groups for a particular purpose can be organized throughout the year, taking into account therapist availability, reduced load during the summer, holidays, and so on. By setting the goal a bit lower than the previous year, it is likely that groups will be filled. Utilization data may provide some obvious target populations to address. Certainly many acute reactive states are likely to recover with limited use of resources. Major depressions and anxiety syndromes require more intensive programming. It is likely that about 15–20% of the clinical population referred to the mental health program will have significant personality disorder features. These patients may need to be managed skillfully or entered into more substantial treatment programs. Special programs for such subgroups as young families, older clients, or specific ethnic populations may be considered.

Programs without special attention to the use of groups often treat less than 5% of their clients in a group format. Relatively straightforward planning as previously described may increase this to 15–20% without too much difficulty. Moving beyond this takes special attention but may be worthwhile. Programs that feature very high levels of group usage are at risk for adverse reactions unless they are very effectively designed and promoted.

(2) Internal Marketing

The value of a group coordinator is revealed in effective marketing of the group program within the service system. This begins with the development of a range of groups that match the needs of the population served. However, groups need to be consistently kept before the eyes of all clinicians who are in a position to refer clients to them. The coordinator must be a visible figure in promoting the use of groups and explaining the rationale for their use. Larger programs may have a weekly group bulletin that lists which groups will be available and when, the number of open slots in these groups, and how to make referrals. Selecting an accurate title for the group is helpful to the referring sources, and a brief description may be made available. Group programs succeed or fail dependent on effective attitudes toward the use of groups by referring sources.

(3) Group Structure

As previously described, the development of a range of groups is necessary to match the needs of the population served. There are strong advantages to the use of groups that are composed on the basis of a common diagnosis or situation. This provides a vehicle for rapid group cohesion and a strong focus on common problems. For the same reasons, closed groups are recommended. Even though the group may have a homogeneous composition in one sense, there is usually plenty of diversity among the members on other characteristics.

Clinical Barriers

(1) Standardized Assessments

A service system is unlikely to be able to stream clients into suitable groups unless a reasonably standardized assessment procedure is in place. This may be achieved by having a subset of clinicians doing all assessments or by having a clear protocol that all clinicians are trained to implement. As previously described, the assessment information can then be applied to a range of groups with clearly defined purposes and composition guidelines. These ideas appear simple in concept but are not easily implemented in a larger system with clinicians of diverse training and experience. The role of the group coordinator is central in ensuring that all assessment clinical staff have the necessary preparation. Ideally, seasoned clinicians are most suitable for the task. Since the smooth functioning of the system is dependent on accurate group assignment, a cursory evaluation by an inexperienced junior staff member is likely to result in dissatisfied clients and therapists alike.

(2) Pretherapy Preparation

The group literature is clear that systematic preparation of potential group members is helpful in getting the group off to a strong start. This reduces the chances of early dropouts who impede group cohesion and may shake motivation. The idea of group preparation might begin with public articles in a newsletter within the plan membership or in the larger media. Clinicians who are assessing and referring clients for group should receive training in how to present to the idea of group and perhaps a handout to give to clients regarding how groups work. Brush off comments about a group's being the only available opening at the moment are sure to discourage members and make them apprehensive about getting involved. It is important that the group therapist have an opportunity to meet with incoming members before they join the group. This meeting has several purposes. It allows a final assessment by the therapist regarding suitability for the particular group being considered. It also provides an opportunity for the therapist to answer questions or concerns about being in a group. Further efforts to identify the focus of therapy can be made. For more specific intensive groups a case can be made for two individual sessions prior to group initiation to accomplish these goals. Above all, the pretherapy meeting begins the development of a therapeutic alliance that helps to sustain the member in the early sessions. Such meetings may not be necessary for psychoeducational groups.

DEVELOPING GROUPS IN SOLO OR SMALL GROUP PRACTICES

Private practitioners today are faced with decreasing referrals and reduced reimbursement for their services. Developing a group program could be professionally and financially rewarding.

The principles outlined in the preceding pages can be applied with some adaptations to the single provider and to small practice groups. The first overriding consideration is to recognize the value of being able to provide both individual and group psychotherapy. Given a rationally designed payment schedule, there should be incentives for both the system and the provider to benefit from greater use of groups. This advantage can be further developed by clearly identifying the general range of diagnoses and problems that can be best served. For a small group practice, this might include some differentiation of function within the clinicians of the group. Such decisions must be connected with a good working knowledge of the types of clients who are served by the referring source. A preliminary discussion, including questions about what problems the system (i.e., managed care organization) is having that need to be addressed, would be helpful. Such discussion also provides an opportunity for input to the system about the most appropriate use of groups. There is likely to be an expansion of services to medically ill patients who are experiencing significant distress or adjustment difficulties.

A program plan that identifies the theoretical models of the groups available (i.e., psychoeducational, cognitive, interpersonal) and the expected number of sessions might then be developed. Such a plan might also outline the advantages of closed groups and some ideas about how often a group could be started. For example, it is likely that a good percentage of referred clients will have depression symptoms. A series of groups for this high-volume diagnosis could be designed. Most clients do not have difficulty with a brief delay when a starting date is specifically scheduled.

Effort should be made to market a therapist's proposal to a managed care organization for the use of groups as a package that includes one or two individual assessment/preparation sessions, a defined number of group sessions, and a follow-up session. For example, two individual sessions, sixteen group sessions of 2 hours duration (including clerical time), plus one follow-up individual session works out to 7 hours per person for an eight member group. This is well within the range for most systems and provides an opportunity for intensive psychotherapy for that portion of the service load requiring more than very brief care.

Most managed care systems are not using groups more regularly because they have not developed a way of implementing them, yet most are quite interested in doing so. Approaching them with a specific plan that might solve their dilemma can be productive. This plan must be couched in terms of specific time limits. The nightmare of a managed care administrator is the thought of an unfocused long-term group, particularly one that might dare to use group process as part of its procedures. Time-limited groups allow a range of models with varying focusing techniques that may or may not employ process emphasis but all within clearly defined utilization patterns. This may require that clinicians obtain further training in adapting to the more stringent requirements of this type of group.

There may also be opportunities to design longer term groups that have primarily a maintenance function—keeping clients out of hospitals and out of emergency rooms, and using fewer primary care visits and medical/diagnostic procedures. Such groups need not necessarily be weekly, but might be biweekly or monthly. Some programs use a flexibly bound group model, in which the group itself meets weekly, but members do not necessarily attend all sessions but rather come as required (Stone 1995). Such groups may have an expanded membership of 20 to 30 clients but a usual group size of 10 or 12. Clients who have severely dysfunctional personality disorders, or those who have a relapsing condition such as severe bipolar disorder or schizophrenia, have found such programs to be of considerable value in decreasing degree and frequency of decompensation episodes.

SUMMARY

The dose–response curve indicates that the great majority of clients respond well to relatively brief psychotherapy. It is useful to distinguish those who present with an acute, often stress-precipitated, condition from those who have a more entrenched set of difficulties. Group formats have been described for each of these clinical populations. Within the time-limited range of a few months, substantial intensive focused psychotherapy can be provided in a cost-effective group format. Several common problem areas that interfere with the development of a comprehensive group program have been identified. Integrated managed care settings offer an opportunity to develop such a program by effectively streaming clients into appropriate groups. Solo or small group practitioners can also design programs for marketing to larger systems utilizing the same principles.

As the managed care field matures, there will be increasing awareness of the value of providing intensive psychotherapy services for clients with more severe and entrenched difficulties. Time-limited groups offer this population an effective format for receiving such clinical care. Indeed, this area of work is becoming increasingly exciting through the development of therapeutic models directed at specific populations. Group psychotherapies are likely to be in increasing demand in the future.

REFERENCES

Barber, J. P., & Crits-Christoph, P. (Eds.). (1995). *Dynamic therapies for psychiatric disorders.* New York: Basic Books.

Beck, A. T., Rush, A. J., & Shaw, B. F., et al. (1979). *Cognitive therapy of depression.* New York: Guilford Press.

Bernard, H. S., & MacKenzie, K. R. (Eds.). (1994). *Basics of group psychotherapy.* New York: Guilford Press.

Crósby, G., & Sabin, J. (1996). Developing and marketing time-limited therapy groups. *Psychiatric Services, 46,* 7–8.

Eysenck, H. J. (1952). The effects of psychotherapy: An evaluation. *Journal of Consulting Psychology, 16,* 319–324.

Fuhriman, A., & Burlingame, G. M. (Eds.). (1994). *Handbook of group psychotherapy: An empirical and clinical synthesis.* New York: Wiley.

Gabbard, G. O., Lazar, S. G., Hornberger, J., & Spiegel, D. (1997). The economic impact of psychotherapy: A review. *American Journal of Psychiatry, 154,* 147–155.

Howard, K. I., Kopta, S. M., Krause, M. S., et al. (1986). The dose–effect relationship in psychotherapy. *American Psychologist, 41,* 159–164.

Kadera, S. W., Lambert, M. J., Andrews, A. A. (1996). How much therapy is really enough: A session-by-session analysis of the psychotherapy dose–response relationship. *Journal of Psychotherapy Practice and Research, 5,* 132–151.

Klerman, G. L., Weissman, M. M., Rounsaville, B. J., et al. (1984). *Interpersonal psychotherapy of depression.* New York: Basic Books.

Kopta, S. M., Howard, K. I., Lowry, J. L., Beutler, L. E. (1994). Patterns of symptomatic recovery in time-unlimited psychotherapy. *Journal of Consulting and Clinical Psychology, 62,* 1009–1016.

Lambert, M. J., Bergin, A. E. (1994). The effectiveness of psychotherapy. In A. E. Bergin & S. L. Garfield (Eds.), *Handbook of psychotherapy and behavior change* (4th ed., pp. 143–189). New York: Wiley.

MacKenzie, K. R. (1994a). Group development. In A. Fuhriman & GM Burlingame GM (Eds.), *Handbook of group psychotherapy* (pp. 223–268). New York: Wiley.

MacKenzie, K. R. (1994). Where is here and when is now? The adaptational challenge of mental health reform for group psychotherapy. *International Journal Group Psychotherapy, 44,* 407–428.

MacKenzie, K. R. (1995). *Effective use of group therapy in managed care.* Washington DC: American Psychiatric Press, Inc.

MacKenzie, K. R. (1996). Time-limited group psychotherapy. Special Section: Termination and group therapy. *International Journal Group Psychotherapy, 46,* 41–60.

MacKenzie, K. R. (Ed.). (1996). The time-limited psychotherapies. In L. J. Dickstein, J. M. Oldham, & M. B. Riba (Eds.), *American psychiatric press review of psychiatry: Vol. 15.* Washington, DC: American Psychiatric Press.

MacKenzie, K. R. (1997a). Clinical application of group development ideas. *Group Dynamics: Theory, Research, and Practice, 1,* 275–287.

MacKenzie, K. R. (1997b). *Time-managed group psychotherapy: Effective clinical applications.* Washington, DC: American Psychiatric Press.

MacKenzie, K. R. (1998). The alliance in time-limited group psychotherapy. In J. D. Safran, & J. C. Muran (Eds.), *The therapeutic alliance in brief psychotherapy* (pp. 193–215). Washington, DC: American Psychological Association.

McKay, M., & Paleg, K. (1992). *Focal group psychotherapy.* Oakland CA: New Harbinger.

National Registry of Certified Group Psychotherapists. (1996). New York, NY: Internal Report: Managed Care Survey.

McRoberts, C., Burlingame, G. M., & Hoag, M. J. (1998). Comparative efficacy of individual and group psychotherapy: A meta-analytic perspective. *Group Dynamics: Theory, Research, and Practice, 2,* 101–117.

Phillips, E. L. (1987). The ubiquitous decay curve: Delivery similarities in psychotherapy, medicine and addiction. *Professional Psychology: Research and Practice, 18,* 650–652.

Piper, W. E., & Joyce, A. S. (1996). A consideration of factors influencing the utilization of time-limited, short-term group therapy. *International Journal of Group Psychotherapy, 46,* 311–328.

Steenbarger, B. N., & Budman, S. H. (1996). Group psychotherapy and managed behavioral health care: Current trends and future challenges. *International Journal of Group Psychotherapy, 46,* 297–309.

Stone, W. N. (1995). *Group psychotherapy for people with chronic illness.* New York: Basic Books.

Tillitski, C. J. (1990). A meta-analysis of estimated effect size for group vs individual vs control treatments. *International Journal of Group Psychotherapy, 40,* 215–224.

Vessey, J. T., Howard, K. I., Lueger, R. J., Kachele, H., & Mergenthaler, E. (1994). The clinician's illusion and the psychotherapy practice: An application of stochastic modeling. *Journal of Consulting and Clinical Psychology, 62,* 679–685.

Winston, A., & Muran, J. C. (1996). Common factors in the time-limited psychotherapies. In L. J. Dickstein, M. B. Riba, & J. M. Oldham (Eds.), *American psychiatric press review of psychiatry, Vol. 15.* Washington, DC: American Psychiatric Press.

Part III

New Roles for Psychologists Under Managed Care

5

The Psychologist
in Primary Health Care

Kirk Strosahl
Mountainview Consulting Group Inc.
Moxee, Washington

As many practicing psychologists can attest, basic political and economic forces are reshaping the mental health delivery system in the United States. This evolution has been stimulated by a growing emphasis on managing how health resources are spent and who receives them. The first generation of managed health care, with its emphasis on cost containment strategies, will soon be accompanied by an intense focus on developing cost *and* quality oriented delivery systems (cf. Cummings, 1995; Strosahl, 1996a, 1997). A key theme in the upcoming era will be the integration of health and behavioral health services. These currently segregated delivery systems will be pressured to merge as a way to reduce redundant administrative and infrastructure costs as well as address consumer demands for simpler "one stop shopping" service delivery venues (Strosahl, 1996b). More fundamentally, integration of services will occur because there is a floor effect in cost oriented health care management strategies, and overly aggressive cost containment strategies can undermine cost, quality, and consumer satisfaction outcomes (Sobel, 1995). There is every indication that purchasers of health care services (primarily government, business, and industry) believe that health care costs cannot be contained as long as health and mental health care are structured as nonoverlapping enterprises. It is now an established fact that medical services utilization is driven by psychological and psychosocial concerns, so much so that effective cost controls requires a redefining of the relationship between health and behavioral health services (Friedman, Sobel, Myers, Caudill, & Banson, 1995).

THE CURRENT PRACTICE ENVIRONMENT AND HOW IT WILL
CHANGE UNDER MANAGED CARE

For decades, psychologists have been trained in an office-based, fee-for-service model of professional specialty practice. In this sense, mental health services have unofficially been "carved out" from health care services. Not surprisingly, guilds such as the American Psychological Association have vigorously opposed the implementation of managed behavioral health care, in much the same way as have medical services guilds. Opponents of the shift to managed care claim that it inappropriately injects financial factors into the process of providing mental health care. This criticism ignores the fact that the fee-for-service, office practice model incorporated into most psychology training programs is itself an economic and business model for providing professional services. In the fee for service model, practitioners make more money by seeing clients for more sessions. This has encouraged borderline clinical practices, such as "diagnosing up" to obtain insurance coverage, problem finding to prolong therapy, and providing long-term therapy for personality reconstruction despite a lack of evidence for the clinical effectiveness or efficacy of such services. Most importantly, the fee-for-service model is responsible for unprecedented increases in insurance premiums. For example, between 1989 and 1994 alone, mental health insurance benefits increased nearly 19% annually (Strosahl, 1994b), a rate far in excess of general inflation. During this period of expansion, the supply of mental health providers of all disciplines grew at astounding rates, to the point that it is likely that the marketplace may be as much as 50% oversupplied with mental health providers. These two factors, uncontrolled annual cost increases and a basic oversupply of providers, provided the opportunity for managed mental health care to evolve in the first place.

In the current practice environment, the financial rules of the road have changed dramatically. With the advent of network provider contracting and at-risk financing models such as capitation, providers make more money by seeing more clients for fewer services. Further, the oversupply of providers has reduced hourly service rates substantially, by as much as 50% in certain areas. There is also a movement to use the lowest capable provider to deliver mental health services, in this case, master's level trained clinicians. Doctoral level psychologists are finding they have a limited niche in most managed care networks, which for the most part make disproportionate use of less expensive master's level providers. Sadly, this means that the clinical services most psychologists have been trained to provide are not in high demand in the mental health specialty marketplace.

To survive and thrive in the managed care environment of the future, psychologists will need to locate new settings for practice, where the clinical need and demand for services is high, and where penetration by other qualified mental health providers is low. As is demonstrated in this chapter, integration of psychological services into primary health care settings carries enormous clinical and financial promise for psychologists willing to make the transition. However, to achieve a meaningful integration, many obstacles need to be overcome, including financing issues, turf struggles, culture clash, and decades of mutual negative stereotyping (Pace, Chaney, Mullins, & Olson, 1995). The most formidable challenge is to provide psychological services that are affordable, practical and consistent with the goals, strategies, and gestalt of primary care medicine.

The purpose of this chapter is to offer psychologists interested in integrating into primary care a specific road map for success. First, epidemiological and services utilization research are explored to highlight not only the tremendous need for mental health services in primary care, but also the impact psychological conditions have on medical services utilization. Second, a primary mental health care model of service delivery is described. Third, the concepts of vertical and horizontal service integration are explored, as they relate to planning and implementing a set of integrated psychological services within a primary care population. Fourth, principles for designing and evaluating medical cost offset programs are articulated. Finally, it will be possible to examine some emerging roles for health psychologists in primary care and how they relate to services provided by other mental health disciplines.

PRIMARY CARE MEDICINE: THE DE FACTO MENTAL HEALTH SYSTEM IN THE UNITED STATES

The *de facto* mental health system in the United States is primary medical care (Reiger et al., 1993). The term "primary care provider" refers to a number of medical disciplines (e.g., family practice, general internal medicine, obstetrics/gynecology, pediatrics) and allied health care specialists (physician's assistants, clinical nurse specialists, registered and licensed nurses, women's health care specialists). Typically, primary care practice is a multidisciplinary team-based enterprise. In the most basic setting, the team is comprised of a single physician and one or more nurses, and frequently other allied health providers in larger practice settings. Each member of the health care team carries out designated functions. In discharging these duties, any team member can encounter patients with mental disorders or significant psychosocial stresses. Research indicates that half of all the formal mental health care in the United States is delivered solely by primary care providers (Narrow, Rae, Manderscheid, & Locke, 1993). Nearly half of all individuals with a diagnosable mental disorder seek no mental health care from any professional, but 80% will visit their primary care physician at least once yearly.

Primary health care providers have been criticized for their poor recognition and treatment of mental disorders and psychosocial issues (Bolestrian, Williams, & Wilkinson, 1988). However, the evidence suggests that most provide both medical and psychosocial interventions to their patients. Nonpsychiatric physicians prescribe approximately 70% of all psychotropic agents, 80% of which are antidepressants (Beardsley, Gardocki, Larson & Hidalgo, 1988). Research into physician–patient interactions reveals that general physicians frequently employ behavioral interventions with their patients (Robinson, 1995a; Robinson et al., 1995). In summary, the existing research suggests that a major role of primary care medicine is that of addressing the psychological needs of the medical patient, often without access to any on-site behavioral health services.

Integration of behavioral health interventions into routine primary care could easily be justified on the basis of the established need for mental health services. However, in the era of managed health care, a more compelling argument arises from evidence about the relationship of psychological distress and medical utilization. Research has shown that a significant proportion of medical visits are generated by symptoms associated with psychological distress or mental disorders (Smith, Rost, & Kashner, 1995). For example, untreated depressed primary care patients use two times the annual medical services as their nondepressed counterparts (Simon, VonKorff, & Barlow, 1995). Another study of the 10 most common physical complaints in primary care revealed that 85% have no diagnosable medical condition during a 3-year follow-up period (Kroenke & Mangelsdorf, 1989).

Studies of physician decision making suggest that only 15–25% of medical decisions are based on health morbidity; the remaining decision making revolves around psychosocial needs, patient preferences, and the doctor–patient relationship (Friedman et al., 1995; Sobel, 1995). As Sobel suggested, there is significant mismatch between the services needed by primary care patients and the services available. This mismatch directly converts into uncontrolled health care utilization. In theory, creation of a better match between patient need and available services should produce better clinical and cost outcomes.

In truth, much of the interest among purchasers in integrating health and behavioral health services is related to the potential for reducing health care costs and, by proxy, insurance premiums. The medical cost offset effect is simply defined as the degree to which health care services are reduced (and costs saved) as a direct consequence of providing behavioral health services instead. Several meta-analyses of studies have examined medical cost offsets achieved through integration of health and behavioral health service. Although the cost offset literature is still in its methodological infancy, various meta-analyses have indicated that provision of behavioral health services to medical patients may result in cost offsets in the range of 20–40% (Friedman et. al., 1995; Sobel, 1995; Strosahl & Sobel, 1996).

POPULATION-BASED CARE: THE MISSION OF PRIMARY CARE

In order to develop and sell integrated behavioral health services, it is critical to understand the philosophy of population-based care and its pivotal role in the primary health care system of today and the future. Population-based care is predicated on a public health approach to services. Rather than focusing on the health of the individual, population-based care emphasizes the importance of processes that address the health and behavioral health care needs of the entire population. A primary care provider's mission is not just to address the health needs of the patient in the office, but to think about similar patients in the population who are part of the physician's "panel." A panel is a cohort of patients and their families who are under the care of a particular physician. A physician carries responsibility not just for treating illness and injury, but also for preventing illness and injury. This leads to fairly central population-based care questions: Are there other patients like this who are not coming in for care? Are there variations in the way services are being provided that result in variable health outcomes? What can prevent conditions from developing in patients who have similar risk factors? Can a consistent process of care that addresses the needs of this patient class in the population we serve be organized?

In order to provide the vast range of clinical services required for effective preventive and palliative care, primary care practice is built to promote a high capacity and high patient turnover rate. In primary care medicine, capacity is created by using 10- to 15-minute visit intervals, so that 30–40 patients can be seen each day. Over the course of a year, this allows up to 80% of all members of a primary care population to have at least one physician visit. This penetration rate into the general population can be contrasted with the 3–4% penetration typically achieved in the specialty mental health system; from this it is easy to draw the conclusion that the mental health system has never adopted a public health, population-based care mission. In a later section, the practice style implications of these different missions becomes all too obvious.

With a wide population penetration, primary care medicine involves treating common causes of medical problems first, then moving to more elaborate medical solutions only if the quicker fix fails. This approach addresses the requirement for rapid turnover, in that on the average, a large percentage of patients respond to general primary treatment strategies. Those who do not respond are quickly moved through an algorithm involving more specialized secondary treatments. If these treatments fail, the patient is no longer seen by the primary care provider, but is referred elsewhere for specialty medical consultations and treatment.

When a framework for integrating behavioral health services into primary care is developed, the same public health perspective applies. For example, what types of behavioral health service needs exist in the population of patients served by this primary care team? What type of service delivery structure allows maximum penetration into the whole population? What types of service interventions work with the common causes of psychological distress? What secondary, and more elaborate, interventions are appropriate for a primary care setting? At what level of complexity is a patient better treated in specialty mental health care? These are pivotal service delivery planning questions. With 80% annual penetration, the "case rate" (i.e., patients who qualify for some form of behavioral health service) is vastly greater in an integrated setting than in a specialty setting, simply because of the volume of patients in the system. Like primary care providers, a psychologist who provides on-site integrated behavioral health needs to use a service approach that allows for high patient volume and high turnover, to address the significantly greater demand for services in the primary care setting. This model must be efficient, yet flexible enough to address a wide array of psychological needs in a way that is valued by primary care team members and consumers. The selection of a workable practice model guarantees a successful transition into primary care settings, but also requires a significant change in clinical philosophy and practice style.

PRIMARY MENTAL HEALTH CARE

Primary mental health care is a consultative practice model that is uniquely suited to the mission, goals, and gestalt of primary care (cf. Quirk et al., 1995; Strosahl, 1994b, 1996b, 1997). In its systemwide application, the primary mental health approach has been determined to be clinically effective and highly acceptable to both primary care providers and consumers (Katon et al., 1996; Robinson, Wischman, & Del Vento, 1996).

Service Philosophies

Numerous service philosophy and practice style features differentiate between primary mental health and specialty mental health care. These differences are summarized in detail elsewhere (Strosahl, 1994b, 1996b, 1997, 1998). The defining service philosophy of the primary mental health care model is to position the psychologist as a behavioral health consultant who is integrated with other primary care team members. Like other members of the team, the psychologist brings specialized knowledge to bear on problems that require behavioral health training and expertise. At the same time, the physician or other health care provider remains in charge of the patient's care. The behavioral health provider may even see the patient for very limited consultative follow-up, but these activities are always designed to support the interventions of the primary care provider. Referrals for behavioral health support can come from any member of the primary care team. Dependent on the practice settings, referrals may predominantly come from physicians, mid-level providers, or nursing staff.

Another pivotal service philosophy difference is the focus on resolving problems within the primary care team structure, rather than on referring all patients to specialty mental health providers. As psychologists integrate with medical practice groups who are engaged in at-risk financing, integrated services will be purchased based on their ability to prevent unnecessary specialty referrals, including to external mental health specialists. Instead, the emphasis will be on managing as many patients as possible and as appropriate within a primary care team.

Whereas effective prevention has been virtually impossible to achieve in specialty mental health systems, it is a central mission of a primary mental health service. Primary care practice involves building and capitalizing on each provider's relationship with the patient over time. This enables the provider to carry the at-risk patient and take a wait-and-see approach without losing contact with the patient. Patients are encouraged to seek health care whenever they are troubled by a physical symptom or when they are seeking a professional opinion about a troubling life circumstance. Preventive behavioral health services function in much the same way. Patients at risk for developing more significant psychological and physical symptoms of distress can be identified and monitored over time by the psychologist providing primary mental health care services.

The Primary Mental Health Care Practice Model

The primary mental health model requires the psychologist to use a consultation model, rather than a specialty therapist model. Most psychologists have less formal training in providing consultative services than in providing direct clinical care. Providing consultation as opposed to therapy services has dramatic practice style implications, which are summarized in Table 5.1. In general, the consultation approach does not involve providing any type of extended treatment services to the patient. The chief customer of the consultation is the patient's primary care provider, not the patient per se. The goal is to help the primary care provider and the patient work most effectively to target and resolve the problems that have arisen in the patient's life. Many consultations are single session visits, with feedback about medication and/or psychological intervention strategies made immediately available to the referring provider. Interventions with patients are simple, bite sized, and compatible with the types of interventions that can be provided in a 15-minute health care visit (i.e., interventions that can be done in 2–3 minutes, maximum). In keeping with the fast pace of primary care practice, consultation visits may be 15–30 minutes in length. The patient is informed that the consultant is being used to help the health care provider and patient come up with an effective plan of attack to target the patient's concerns. When called for, follow-up consultative visits are designed to reinforce and build on the health care provider's interventions. The goal is to maximize over time what often amounts to a very limited number of visits to either the consultant or the health care provider. Thus, the consultant is able to follow patients who need longer term surveillance "at an arm's length," in a manner that is very consistent with how primary care providers manage their at-risk patients. As previously mentioned, the primary care physician/provider is still responsible for choosing, implementing, and monitoring the results of interventions. In the primary mental health model, the consultant can provide an extensive number of clinical services. These may include assistance with treatment planning and monitoring, patient education classes, relapse prevention, and team building to name a few.

TABLE 5.1

Features Distinguishing Primary Mental and Specialty Mental Health Services

Dimension	Primary mental health	Specialty mental health
1. Service goals	1. Support provider interventions 2. Improve provider interventions 3. Teach provider core clinical skills 4. Educate patient in self- management skills through exposure 5. Improve provider–patient relationship 6. Monitor at-risk patients 7. Support management of chronic cases by provider 8. Assist in primary care team building	1. Deliver primary treatment to resolve condition 2. Coordinate with primary care provider only as needed 3. Teach patient core mental health skills 4. Manage more serious mental disorder over time as primary provider
2. Referral structure	1. Referral by provider	1. Patient self-refers/referred by others
3. Session structure	1. Limited to one to three visits in typical case 2. 15- to 30-minute visits	1. Session number variable, related to index condition 2. 50-minute hour

continued on next page

4. Treatment structure	1. Informal, revolves around provider referral question 2. Long between-session interval 3. Relationship generally not primary focus 4. Visits timed around provider visits 5. Long-term follow-up rare; reserved for high risk cases	1. Formal, requires intake assessment, treatment planning 2. Short between-session interval 3. Relationship key goal over time 4. Visit structure unrelated to medical visits 5. Long-term follow-up encouraged for most clients
5. Intervention strategies	1. Limited 1:1 visit 2. Uses patient education model as primary model 3. Consultant is a technical resource to patient 4. Emphasis on home-based practice to promote change 5. May involve provider in visits with patient	1. One-to-one contact is primary modality 2. Education adjunctive strategy to therapy 3. Therapist directs change strategies 4. Homework linked back to treatment 5. Provider not involved in visits with patient
6. Case Completion	1. Responsibility returned to provider in toto 2. Provider provides relapse prevention or maintenance treatment	1. Therapist retains primary provider role 2. Therapist provides relapse prevention or maintenance treatment
7. Documentation	1. Consultation report to provider 2. Part of medical record	1. Intake report or session progress note 2. Part of mental health chart

Note. "Provider" refers to any primary health care provider including physician, physician's assistant, clinical nurse specialist, registered nurse, licensed practical nurse, woman's health care specialist, etc.

A major feature of the consultative services approach is that it allows *in vivo* training to occur, built around specific casework. Over time, with feedback about hundreds of patients sent to the consultant, health care providers gain direct experience using effective diagnostic and treatment strategies. The knowledge that there is an on-site consultant to provide support often frees primary care providers to engage in new interventions that previously would not have been feasible in an unsupported practice setting. Eventually, primary care providers integrate the skills, and implement both psychological and pharmacological interventions more effectively.

CORE PRACTICE STYLE ISSUES

It should be obvious that primary mental health care is a unique type of clinical service that requires a different set of skills and practice style adaptations. In addition, the realities of the primary care setting make further demands on the clinical practice style of the consultant. This section is examines the most important issues effecting clinical practice in this new model.

Do Not Become the House Shrink

The traditional therapist role, even if it involves brief therapy, is not a viable option in applied primary care settings. There are numerous disadvantages associated with becoming the "house shrink," not the least of which is that most medical practice groups are unwilling or unable to pay for on-site specialty mental health services. Even if funding were available, the level of manifest need in primary care settings would completely outstrip the capacity of the mental health provider. This would quickly lead to access problems for new physician referrals and the accumulation of a variety of chronic, multiproblem patients who never leave therapy, whether it is provided in a specialty mental health clinic or in a primary care center. In other words, the psychologist would quickly revert back to providing services that were inconsistent with a population-based care framework. Consultation experience with systems that have tried to use the house shrink model suggests that mental health providers quickly become marginal members of the primary care team. Ironically, the therapist role actually reinforces the stereotypic separation of health and mental health services by encouraging primary care providers to transfer responsibility for managing mental health issues. Given the frequency with which primary care services involve discussing psychosocial and mental health issues, this is an unhealthy message to give to primary care team members.

The 30-Minute Hour

To fit in with the gestalt of primary care, it is necessary to evaluate and make recommendations rapidly, normally within a 30-minute visit time frame. This may often occur without a chart and, in some cases, without a specific referral question. How can this be done in a way that produces quality outcomes from the physician and patient perspective?

First, consultative services are designed to support the physician's ongoing interventions with the patient. It is not necessary to develop an elaborate assessment or treatment plan to build positive momentum. A prime example is the capturing of an elaborate psychosocial, treatment, and family history. This consumes a great deal of time in an initial visit, but just how relevant is it to forming one or two recommendations for a physician who knows the patient better than the consultant in the first place? This does not mean the consultant ignores information in these areas. However, experience suggests that most relevant information occurs spontaneously when the focus is on current functioning and behavior change. A typical primary mental health visit has the following structure: (a) spend 2–3 minutes with introductions and links back to the physician, (b) spend 5–10 minutes getting a sense of the problem from the patient, and (c) spend 15 minutes generating one or two specific behavioral interventions and forming a follow-up plan.

The Gestalt of Primary Care

Psychologists intent on practicing in primary care need to appreciate the profound difference between the atmosphere of primary care and that of specialty mental health care. When patients enter a doctor's office, they expect to be prodded, poked, measured, advised, handed pamphlets, and asked to do something to address a medical problem or improve general physical health (e.g., cut down on eating fats, see the diabetes educator, etc.). In other words, the primary care environment is characterized by action, advice, and directives. In contrast, patients who enter psychotherapy are hoping that things will change for the better but believe that talking about the possibilities of, and obstacles to, potential change is first required. When patients cross the "mental health threshold,", their vision of what it takes to reach a solution changes with them. This makes specialty mental health work different in its emphasis on persuasion and rapport building. In essence, the mental health setting is not action oriented.

The immediate implications of this difference are that (a) the rules governing patient provider interactions in primary care are substantially different, and (b) primary care patients are ready to be advised and directed, without requiring all the verbal manipulations of therapy. A major practice style change associated with this is that it is acceptable to be blunt about discussing problems and directing behavior change. For example, it is completely acceptable to advise a patient experiencing panic attacks as follows: "I would like you to practice breathing regularly for at least 15 minutes a day, once in the morning and once in the evening. I want you to let your doctor know how the practice is going when you see him or her next week." These action-oriented directives seldom work in psychotherapy, without a significant amount of rationale giving and discussion. In primary care, the patient *expects* to leave with a set of recom-

mended actions. A distinctive feature of primary care work is the degree of
change that can be achieved with a minimum of effort. Comparing minute for
minute spent, the psychologist consultant has a far greater impact on symptom
reduction and behavior change than he or she does in specialty mental health.

The power to dramatically effect clinical outcomes by providing minimal
consultative structure is illustrated in the Integrated Care Program for Depression, which employs a combination of doctor and behavioral health consultant
visits to treat depressed primary care patients (Robinson et al., 1996). In approximately 3–4 hours total treatment time, this type of intervention program
produced therapeutic effect sizes comparable or superior to field studies that
employed 16–20 hours of specialty mental health care (Katon et al., 1996).

Differentiate Consultation From Therapy

Another significant issue in primary care mental health is that of ensuring the
patient and physician understand the goals and objectives of consultation, and
how these might differ from the goals of psychotherapy. In most cases, patients
have little trouble understanding this distinction and do not have rigid precon-
ceptions about what type of behavioral health support is helpful. In addition, by
avoiding any references to therapy and correcting the patient's labeling of consultation as therapy, the consultant can work with the patient using a set of mu-
tually agreed on parameters. In almost any primary care practice, there will be
at least one physician/provider who wants to use the consultant to provide therapy to his or her most frustrating or intractable patients. Although primary care
providers frequently access consultative specialists for medical help, they have
no particular history like this with psychologists. In most cases, they carry a
very specific stereotype about the practice of mental health that includes psychotherapy and the 50-minute hour. Although typical primary care providers
can easily identify with the goals and strategies of primary care medicine, they
normally do not associate this with mental health providers and so need help in
learning about this new role. The clearer this initial impression is for the patient
and referring provider, the less likely it is that misunderstandings will develop
about the role of the psychologist.

Learn to Address Medication Issues

A primary mental health psychologist must be able to competently and confi-
dently discuss medication questions with patients and/or referring health care
providers. As noted earlier, 80% of all psychotropic medications are prescribed
by general physicians. Frequently, the primary care provider refers a patient with
two goals in mind: one is to start some type of behavioral health intervention; the
second is to hear the consultant's opinion as to whether the patient is on the right
medication or can profit from starting a medication. Normally, this involves antidepressants and benzodiazapines, the two drugs prescribed most often by general physicians. It is hard to be effective in the consultant role without being

conversant about the thinking, feeling, and behavioral effects of psychotropic medications. Any psychologist intent on integrating into primary care should learn about the various classes of medication, to know their generic and trade names, their side effects, doses and titration, and potentially dangerous drug–drug interactions. The psychologist needs to understand and communicate that the decision to prescribe or not prescribe, to change medications or their dosage, remains the sole responsibility of the provider with prescriptive authority. The psychologist consultant assists with general information about the efficacy of medication treatment for particular conditions and which medication classes seem to achieve the best outcomes, based on the available research.

For example, seratonin reuptake inhibitors (SRIs) such as Prozac and Paxil are widely prescribed for dysthymia, subthreshold depressive symptoms, and major depression. SRIs are usually favored by general physicians because of their innocuous side-effect profiles, which result in fewer unplanned follow-up visits to address patient concerns. In addition, physicians receive an overwhelming amount of marketing literature on antidepressants, which leads to the tendency to overprescribe antidepressants in general, and SRIs in particular. Physicians are less likely to know that evidence suggests antidepressants are no better than drug placebos with subthreshold conditions with specialty mental health patients and that they do not seem to make much of a difference in the treatment of minor depression among primary care patients (Katon et al., 1996).

Obviously, the primary care mental health provider must know the literature on the clinical efficacy of medications, alternatives to medication treatment, and differential diagnostic considerations. To develop this knowledge, the consultant should read texts on drug therapy written for nonmedical practitioners, stay abreast of the psychiatric literature on the clinical efficacy of new and established agents, and participate in continuing education workshops where possible. It is imperative that the consultant understand the limits of his or her competence in this area and, when called for, refer the patient and provider to an appropriately trained professional.

DEVELOPING INTEGRATED BEHAVIORAL HEALTH SERVICES: HORIZONTAL AND VERTICAL INTEGRATION APPROACHES

Psychologists are in a unique position to develop, implement, and evaluate integrated primary mental health services in primary care. However, the gestalt of primary care is fast paced and chaotic, and the need for services far outstrips the supply. This requires systematic program and service planning based on population-based care principles. Psychologists who take the time to assess population demographics, met and unmet needs, and cost effectiveness stand the best chance of successfully marketing their services to primary care practice groups. In general, there are two program planning philosophies that can be used individually or in combination.

Horizontal integration involves providing services designed to impact the behavioral health needs of the entire primary care population. The generic behavioral health consultation model described earlier is a textbook example of a horizontally integrated service. A distinguishing feature of horizontal integration is that it casts a wide net in terms of how it defines health care needs and how it defines the population to be served. Traditional primary care medicine is largely based on the horizontal integration approach. The provider delivers a wide array of services across his or her panel, with the goal of improving the health and well being of the entire cohort of patients under his or her care. In this approach, every member of the panel is encouraged to have a primary care visit. Different services are provided to patients based on unique needs but, in the aggregate, regular visits from most panel members allow the primary care provider to "tend the flock." Horizontal integration is the platform on which all other forms of integrated behavioral health care reside, because many members of the primary care population can benefit from a generic psychological consultation.

Vertical integration involves providing targeted behavioral health services to a well-defined, circumscribed group of primary care patients. This is a major contemporary development in primary care medicine and behavioral health as well. Vertical integration programs usually target high-frequency and/or high-cost patient populations such as depression, panic disorder, chemical dependency and certain groups of high medical utilizers. A complaint that frequently occurs in a given population, such as depression, is a good candidate for a special process of care. Some conditions, although rare in the general population, are so costly that they require a special system of care. In the behavioral health arena, chronic pain patients are a small but costly group who often are the targets of vertical integration programs (Strosahl & Sobel, 1996). The core strategy for psychologists using a vertical integration approach is to develop systematic screening, care management, and relapse prevention protocols that integrate the activities of the psychologist and primary care providers into a single coherent "pathway." In addition, the psychologist can develop a program evaluation component that allows patient outcomes to be tracked, so that physicians can see the benefits of working collaboratively with a consulting psychologist. A classic example of the clinical pathway approach is the integrated care program for depression (Robinson et al., 1996), which is designed for primary care patients with major and minor depression.

DEVELOPMENT OF VERTICAL AND HORIZONTAL PROGRAMS TO ACHIEVE COST OFFSETS

A major stimulus for integrating health and behavioral health services is the potential for medical cost savings. In general, psychologists interested in providing integrated services should be knowledgeable about the medical cost offset literature and understand the mechanisms that produce offsets (cf. Sobel, 1995). Briefly, the major cost offset mechanisms are as follows:

1. Information and decision-support pathway: Empowers patients with safe, effective self-care and self-management strategies.
2. Psycholophysiological stress response pathway: Decrease the chronic, inappropriate physiological stress response.
3. Lifestyle or behavior change pathway: Support successful behavior change strategies to decrease health-damaging behaviors and increase health-promoting behaviors.
4. Social support pathway: Increase perceived levels of social support and reduce social isolation.
5. Psychiatric disorder pathway: Improve the detection and treatment of unrecognized psychiatric conditions.
6. Somatization pathway: Identify physical symptoms that are expressions of emotional distress and help patients develop alternative coping strategies.

Any of these mechanisms may singly or in combination elevate medical utilization. In most cases, these mechanisms are well suited to simple, targeted screening and intervention procedures. This information is critical in designing specific programs that may be of clinical and financial interest to primary care practice groups. How can the learnings from the cost offset literature be applied in primary care settings? What are the ingredients for success? Table 5.2 presents specific cost offset target populations and some sample programs that have been designed and implemented to achieve cost offsets.

BASIC PRINCIPLES IN COST OFFSET PROGRAM DESIGN

Because of the extensive number of behavioral health services that could be delivered in primary care, it is important to plan programs that deliver the greatest "punch for the buck." In many cases, the degree of cost offset achieved in a demonstration program directly influences whether a primary care group will contract for even more integrated psychological services. The following principles are offered to help psychologists be successful in demonstrating and capitalizing on medical cost offset potential.

Select the Right Population

When developing cost offset programs, it always advisable to recall the following cardinal rule of vertical integration: Identify the high-cost, high-prevalence conditions, situations, and patient populations in which there is reason to believe a cost-effective intervention exists or can be developed. For example, many health maintenance organizations have focused their attention on treating depression in primary care because (a) it is very prevalent in the general medical and specialty mental health population, and (b) in its untreated form, it is associated with very high medical utilization. In this case, the cost offset mechanism being targeted is the "psychiatric disorder pathway."

TABLE 5.2
Cost Offset Pathways and Corresponding Integrated Service Programs

Cost offset pathway	General behavioral consultation model (horizontal integration)	Clinical pathway response (vertical integration)
Information, support, and self-management	Distribute informational brochures about a wide variety of health and behavioral health conditions; prescribe self-help reading; attempt to normalize adjustment issues; help patients focus on feasible, practical coping responses that can be reinforced during PCP visits; use periodic booster visits to increase motivation, skill refinement	Classroom model services providing information on such issues as living with chronic illness, returning to work from disability, and general health and nutrition skills; provide specialized education and telephone support around disease-specific self-management skills (e.g., diabetes self-monitoring)
Psycho-physiologic stress response	Teach core stress management skills (i.e., regular exercise, taking breaks, time management, breathing retraining), use home-based practice, help PCP make decisions regarding medication management of physical symptoms, use strategic spacing of follow-up consultation visits, coordinate on-the-job coping skills with employer	Longer lasting class or group on stress management and relaxation strategies, expose participants to wide range of coping skills, build education modules that can address specific stress issues including health and behavioral health conditions, help patients develop individually tailored stress management goals
Social support	Try to help patient build linkages with community supports, provide infrequent but predictable consultation visits to deflect social support seeking, distribute planned support across primary care team, help avoid use of unneeded antianxiety/antidepressant agents	Implement weekly group care clinics for at-risk patients with organized social support context and a combination of behavioral health and medical providers, provide manual-based telephone support by nursing staff, provide field-based nursing home "rounding" services

continued on next page

Lifestyle change/ health risk	Help patient formulate specific goals that can be monitored during health care visits, help primary care team members avoid counter-instructional pressure, help isolate and treat co-morbid behavior disorders that interfere with progress	Offer specific behavior change curricula such as smoking cessation and weight reduction, offer structured lifestyle change support using phone boosters, help monitor co-occurring medical interventions such as nicotine replacement
Psychiatric disorder	Help with differential diagnosis for primary care provider, provide with doable behavior change interventions, help assess need for medication, educate patient about side effects and compliance issues, provide strategic follow ups to reinforce behavior change, provide support for relapse prevention planning and/or medication tapering	Implement disorder specific program such as integrated care program for depression, provide self-management skill-building program suited to individual or classroom format, adopt a temporary co-management arrangement with primary care provider, use workbook approach such as Living life well: New strategies for hard times (Robinson,1996)
Somatization	Help create linkage between stress and somatization symptoms, help primary care team avoid confrontations around mind–body dichotomy, provide individual biofeedback and relaxation training, help patient with distorted cognitive interpretations of somatic symptoms, help primary care team develop utilization management plan	Implement longer classroom or group program for high utilizing,somaticizing patients using structured workbook approach, including exposure to stress-somatization linkage concepts and tailoring education modules to allow for customized goal setting; see Healthy mind, healthy body workbook (Sobel &Ornstein, 1996), for example

Develop Accurate Screening/Entry Procedures

When developing a cost offset program, make sure that the eligible target population is clearly defined and that any screening or program entry procedures produce accurate results. For example, it is very difficult to realize optimal cost offsets among the depressed population without an accurate method for detecting depression. Use of unclear criteria or poor screening tools results in ineligible patients being included in interventions and eligible patients being excluded. Each of these outcomes lowers the net potential for achieving offsets.

Match the Intervention with the Mechanism

Any intervention program needs to target one or more of the hypothesized cost offset mechanisms. The corresponding risk is to build an intervention that creates a mismatch. For example, a program for high utilizing older patients with minor symptoms of depression might incorrectly focus on medical and/or therapeutic treatment of depression. If the more basic mechanism is social isolation or disenfranchisement, the program runs the risk not only of being clinically ineffective, but actually driving up medical costs as well, due to the use of expensive new generation antidepressant medicines. Although this principle seems obvious in theory, it is difficult in application, particularly when a targeted population exhibits multiple cost offset mechanisms.

Create Structured Program Materials

Very often, psychologists are in consulting relationships with several primary care sites. These sites may be part of a larger multispecialty practice network. This creates the need to develop and implement interventions that minimize variation among providers and sites. Clinical interventions organized around best practices are more efficient, are easier to evaluate, and produce more consistent quality health outcomes. Turning providers loose on a population without an overarching structure will lead to greater variation in treatment costs and outcomes. Remember, the achieved cost offset is the difference between the cost to treat using behavioral health services and the resulting reduction in medical costs. Frequently, materials can be structured to provide both a provider treatment manual and patient education workbooks. This allows the psychologist to train primary care team members in administration of a classroom, group, or individual program. The integrated program for depression is an excellent example of this highly structured, manual- and workbook-based approach (Robinson et al., 1996).

BASIC PRINCIPLES IN DEMONSTRATING COST OFFSETS

As previously discussed, a major challenge to implementing integrated behavioral health services lies in convincing medical decision makers to buy into the cost offset argument. In this situation, the psychologist becomes a "program evaluator," using the research training that is commonplace in most training programs. However, evaluating cost offsets is unlike other, more straightforward clinical research, because it involves capturing clinical outcome, service utilization, and cost data. At the same time, many of the rules of controlled clinical research still apply. Understanding the following evaluation guidelines will help ensure that cost offsets can be detected.

Measure Cost Effectiveness and Cost Offset

Although it is tempting to look strictly at medical cost reductions alone, this can sometimes create a misleading picture. For example, cost offsets can be achieved by reducing the cost of the index interventions or by reductions in general medical utilization that occur after the intervention. An extremely inexpensive and less robust intervention program can produce an immediate cost offset, but in the long run may actually increase costs due to higher relapse rates, deterioration in self-management efficacy, and so forth. A novel approach to demonstrating medical cost offset is to measure the cost effectiveness of an integrated behavioral health intervention program in comparison with usual medical care, which may involve referring a patient for specialty mental health services. This approach looks at both reduced medical costs and the direct costs and clinical outcomes associated with providing specialized programmatic treatment. One study conducted at Group Health Cooperative showed that an integrated treatment program for depression achieved an incremental cost effectiveness of $940 per patient treated, as compared to usual medical and mental health care (Von Korff et al., in press). These results suggest that demonstrating incremental cost effectiveness on a case-by-case basis may be a more powerful method of demonstrating the financial viability of a cost offset program.

Establish Baseline Costs

To demonstrate a cost offset, it is first necessary to establish the baseline cost to treat a target population in terms of both behavioral health services and medical services. A solid, stable estimate of the baseline medical costs for a target population must be available prior to the initiation of a cost offset program.

Capture All Pertinent Costs

A proper measurement of offsets requires an estimate of not only direct service costs (i.e., direct behavioral health services, medical visits, and procedures) but also ancillary services (lab, pharmacy, ER services, specialty consultations, and procedures) and indirect services (community home health, visiting nurse, nursing home liaison, or support). It can be a fatal marketing error to underestimate the degree of savings by failing to capture all of the service costs required to treat a population. In addition to direct medical costs, it is also advisable to include indirect costs such as work absenteeism, turnover, and lost productivity. Medical practice groups will be under increasing pressure from employer purchasers to demonstrate positive impacts on worker health and productivity. Integration of data sources such as these will only make a cost offset program more likely to receive ongoing support.

Develop Realistic Service Costs

Behavioral health and medical services differ not only in the direct cost to pay providers, but also in the overhead required to support the service delivery environment. For example, a physician visit not only involves the doctor, but also requires nursing support, medical equipment and supplies, and so on. When a cost estimate of a physician or behavioral health visit is being developed, these overhead factors need to be included. Otherwise, the cost to treat may be overestimated and the cost of usual care will be deflated. The result is that there is a smaller than expected cost offset.

Measure the Nuclear Family

Failure to track medical utilization in a patient's family can create a misleading medical offset picture. In certain target populations (e.g., alcohol abuse) cost offsets can be most strongly associated with decreased medical utilization among family members of patients. Improvement in the physical and psychological health of the patient may well reduce the stress and burden of caregiving among immediate family members, which in turn reduces their tendency to use medical services to remedy stress-related issues.

Select an Appropriate Time Frame

Although some programs have achieved cost offsets within a matter of hours (in the case of presurgical preparation) to months, other interventions may require 1–3 years to fully realize cost offsets. It is not unusual for cost offsets to accelerate over a 2- to 3-year period. This is probably due to the fact that behavioral health interventions first impact the patient's general sense of well-being followed by a reduction in symptoms. However, changes in general functioning and patterns of medical utilization tend to occur much more slowly, often after clinical symptoms have been absent for months. In addition, certain relapse prone conditions accumulate medical cost offsets by cycling through the relapse risk corridor without incident, thus saving direct treatment costs that have to be delivered to the untreated control group. Depression is an excellent example of such a condition.

Use an Appropriate Control Group

Over time, high utilizers of medical services will tend to drift back to the center of the utilizer curve. Because of regression to the mean, demonstration of a cost offset requires a control group of similar patients who are not exposed to the intervention program. Ideally, patients can be randomly assigned to the "new program" or to "usual care." Practically speaking, wait list controls are not feasible in the primary care setting. The best alternative control group is usual care, specifically, a matched group of patients who are allowed to receive medical services as usual, but are not allowed to enroll in the cost offset program.

EMERGING ROLES FOR THE HEALTH PSYCHOLOGIST IN PRIMARY CARE

Psychologists, by virtue of their unique training background, have a great deal to offer within a typical primary care setting. Throughout this chapter, the reader has been exposed to a primary mental health practice model as well as a template for integrative program design and evaluation. Table 5.3 summarizes basic aspects of the psychologist's role in the ideal primary care team environment. As is seen, some services provided by doctoral level psychologists are unique and do not overlap with those provided by master's level providers. On the other hand, other general services might be provided by any appropriately trained behavioral health provider. Although it is certainly advisable for psychologists interested in integration to offer general services, the market niche for psychology in the integrated care system of the future will probably involve the provision of services that are less likely to be delivered by competing disciplines.

In order for psychologists to market their services effectively to primary care practice groups, it is useful to examine some new and emerging service needs that may be well suited to the practice of psychology. The basis for these projections is the anticipation that the health care market place will be pressured to integrate services and develop direct financial relationships between purchasers and providers.

The Psychologist as Mid-level Provider

Although there is an ongoing and heated controversy about whether to allow psychologists prescriptive authority, there is little doubt that a doctoral level behavioral health specialist equipped with prescription privileges would be an extremely valuable commodity in primary care. A major contemporary trend in primary care is the use of "provider extender" professionals such as nurse practitioners, physician's assistants, and so forth. This approach creates more cost efficiency by allowing such mid-level providers to provide routine health care, reserving more expensive physician time for truly complicated health issues. The prescribing psychologist would fill a natural void in the primary care setting. Rather than the team physician directing routine medication treatment, the psychologist would be given that responsibility. The ability to integrate appropriate psychological and pharmacological treatment within a single provider could have an enormous impact on the quality of behavioral health care.

TABLE 5.3
Major Service Roles for Psychologists in Integrated Primary Care Settings

Service type	Definition
1. Behavioral health consultation	Service for patient referred for a general evaluation; focus on diagnostic and functional evaluation, recommendations for treatment, and forming limited behavior change goals; involves assessing patients at risk because of some life stress event; may involve limited follow-up contacts
2. Integrated program consultation	Uses manual-based condensed specialty patient education package conducted by the consultant; visit usually linked to planned provider visits; involves four to six short sessions of temporary comanagement; usually part of critical pathway program for mental condition such as depression, panic disorder, or somatization
3. Specialty consultation	Service designed to support management of chronically distressed, high utilizing patients; visits provided at predictable long intervals over time; often part of team-based medical management plan to control excessive unscheduled medical visits
5. Conjoint consultation	Service for physician and patient designed to address an issue of concern to both; often involves addressing a conflict in the working relationship about diagnosis, treatment, or compliance issues
6. On demand consultation	Service provided to help address emergent cases encountered during daily medical practice; may involve phone or face-to-face contact; consultant may be available on site or by paging system, best if on site
7. Medication management	Service goal is to help patient comply with medication initiated by provider; focus on education, addressing negative beliefs, or strategies for coping with side effects; may help prescribers comply with medication practice guidelines
8. Relapse prevention	Service goal is to maintain treatment gains for patient who has responded to medication/psychosocial treatment; uses booster session strategy over time; often involves monitoring medication tapering at request of physician

continued on next page

9. Behavioral medicine	Service for patients who must learn to manage chronic medical illness; may be used to help patients tolerate invasive or uncomfortable medical procedures; focus may be on lifestyle issues or health risk factors among patients at risk (e.g., smoking cessation, post myocardial infarction behavior change)
10. Disability management	Service goal is to assist physician in managing work disability for behavioral health or combined conditions; coordinate treatment services and work with employer to develop effective return to work plan; may also involve assisting with initial disability determination
11. Occupational health	Service goal is to provide behavioral health evaluations for worker's compensation claims; includes coordinating treatment services for chronic pain injuries, developing return-to-work group or class, and acting as an agent in the claims adjudication process
13. Chronic pain	Service goal is to provide assistance to physicians managing chronic pain patients on site; includes developing program for pain management skills and assisting in the acute phase management new pain complaints

The Psychologist as Population Manager

As population-based care broadens its foothold as the dominant health care service philosophy, the psychologist in primary care will be in the unique and enviable position of engaging in true primary prevention. Psychologists not only will provide specialized consultation and programmatic services for patients who already have problems, but also will monitor routine behavioral health in much the same way physicians provide "well visits" and protocol-based preventive services (e.g., immunizations, breast cancer screening). In population based care parlance, the psychologist will act as the behavioral health "population manager." Given a population manager approach, a large percentage of behavioral health visits should be well visits, or routine behavioral health checkups that would allow at risk patients to be identified and monitored over time. Whereas prescription privileges would initiate a major structural change for the psychologist in primary care, the role of population manager would precipitate a major transition in service philosophy.

The Psychologists as Occupational Health Provider

As employer purchasers and medical practice groups continue the current trend of direct, at-risk contracting, a major shift in the focus of primary care medi-

cine will occur. There will be an increased emphasis on functional health outcomes such as missed work days, lost work productivity, and functional
disability. This will occur primarily because the purchasers want to see more
direct benefits of employer-subsidized medical care in the workplace. Currently, employers spend approximately 8% of their total revenues on
short-term disability insurance (Strosahl & Johnson, in press). There is a
widely held belief in business that disability and occupational health issues are
not being systematically and effectively addressed in the health care system.
Medical practice groups that offer value-added disability prevention and management services will have a competitive advantage in the marketplace.

Effective occupational health and disability management requires as much
attention to behavioral health issues as it does to physical medicine. The psychologist working in primary care has an important role to play in addressing
the behavioral aspects of occupational medicine. Normally, this means the psychologist must collaborate with physicians to minimize the iatrogenic potential of some medical treatments (e.g., the use of narcotic analgesics with fresh
back injury patients) and maintain or restore the patient's functional capacity
so that a quick return to work can occur. Psychologists practicing in primary
care need to learn how the short-term disability and worker's compensation
systems function and acquire skills for the management of functional disability
(Strosahl & Johnson, in press).

SUMMARY

In this chapter, we have examined how managed behavioral health care is both
depriving psychologists of certain traditional job opportunities and promoting a
host of new ones. Primary care medicine is the *de facto* mental health system in
the United States, yet there are only a handful of primary care systems that have
any form of integrated behavioral health services. This truly represents the single
largest opportunity for psychologists to prosper in the next millennium.

Working in primary care as a behavioral clinician requires much effort and
many practice style adjustments, so it is quite understandable that clinicians
ask, "What's in it for me?" Apart from job security in an increasingly competitive practice environment, there are numerous other benefits. In my experience, the most rewarding aspect has been the tremendous value attached to
primary mental health services by members of the primary care team. The primary care setting is desperately lacking in access to behavioral health services
and, to no small extent, a behavioral health consultant is something of a local
hero. Interventions that seem simple and just a matter of common sense to a
well-trained behavioral clinician are often viewed as minor miracles by primary care providers.

From a clinical perspective, a second reward comes in experiencing the dramatic positive effects of integrated health and mental health care. Because of
the enormous need for services, the primary care context provides a much
broader forum for the provision of psychological services. Although specialty

mental health work is interesting, there is nowhere near the diversity of problems and opportunities for solutions that are available in primary care. For example, meaningful preventive care is almost impossible in the specialty mental health settings, but in primary care it is a feasible, culturally acceptable service. Patients who would never visit a psychotherapist can nevertheless receive useful psychological services.

Perhaps the most significant reward is the personal and professional growth that occurs when working in a blended context that integrates mind and body medicine. I have experienced both personal and professional growth as a result of seeing primary care providers as human beings, not as stereotypes. The vast majority of health care providers have a deep commitment to helping others and an equally deep sense of remorse when the outcome is bad. This leads to a much greater appreciation of the major role physical health and medicine can and does play in promoting the patient's overall sense of well-being. With the integration of health and behavioral health, there is an excellent opportunity for practicing psychologists to influence treatment of the whole person.

REFERENCES

Beardsley, R., Gardocki, G., Larson, D., & Hidalgo, J. (1988). Prescribing of psychotropic medication by primary care physicians and psychiatrists. *Archives of General Psychiatry, 45,* 1117–1119.

Bolestrian, S., Williams, P., & Wilkinson, G. (1988). Specialist mental health treatment in general practice: A meta-analysis. *Psychological Medicine, 18,* 711–717.

Cummings, N. (1995). Impact of managed care on employment and training: A primer for survival. *Professional Psychology: Research and Practice, 26,* 10–15.

Friedman, R., Sobel, D., Myers, P., Caudill, M., & Benson, H. (1995). Behavioral medicine, clinical health psychology and cost offset. *Health Psychology, 14,* 509–518.

Katon, W., Robinson, P., Von Korff, M., Lin, E., Bush, T., Ludman, E., Simon, G., & Walker, E. (1996). A multifaceted intervention to improve treatment of depression in primary care. *Archives of General Psychiatry, 53,* 924–932.

Kroenke, K., & Mangelsdorf, A. (1989). Common symptoms in primary care: Incidence, evaluation, therapy and outcome. *American Journal of Medicine, 86,* 262–266.

Narrow, W. Reiger, D., Rae, D., Manderscheid, R., & Locke, B. (1993). Use of services by persons with mental and addictive disorders: Findings from the National Institute of Mental Health Epidemiologic Catchment Area Program. *Archives of General Psychiatry, 50,* 95–107.

Pace, T., Chaney, J., Mullins, L & Olson, R. (1995). Psychological consultation with primary care physicians: Obstacles and opportunities in the medical setting. *Professional Psychology: Research and Practice, 26,* 123–131.

Quirk, M., Strosahl, K., Todd, J., Fitzpatrick, W., Casey, M., Hennessey, S., & Simon, G. (1995). Quality and customers: Type 2 change in mental health delivery within health care reform. *Journal of Mental Health Administration, 22,* 414–425.

Reiger, D., Narrow, W., Rae, D., Manderschied, R., Locke, B., & Goodwin, F. (1993). The de facto US mental and addictive disorders service system: Epidemiologic Catchment Area prospective 1 year prevalence rates of disorders and services. *Archives of General Psychiatry, 50,* 85–94.

Robinson, P. (1995). New territory for the behavior therapist: Hello depressed patients in primary care! *The Behavior Therapist, 18,* 145–153.

Robinson, P., Bush, T., Von Korff, M., Katon, W., Lin, E., Simon, G., & Walker, E. (1995). Primary care physician use of cognitive behavioral techniques with depressed patients. *Journal of Family Practice, 40,* 352–357.

Robinson, P., Wischman, C., & Del Vento, A. (1996). *Treating depression in primary care: A manual for physicians and therapists.* Reno, NV: Context Press.

Simon, G., VonKorff, M., & Barlow, W. (1995). Health care costs of primary care patients with recognized depression. *Archives of General Psychiatry, 52,* 850–856.

Smith, G., Rost, K., & Kashner, T. (1995). A trial of the effect of a standardized psychiatric consultation on health outcomes and costs in somaticizing patients. *Archives of General Psychiatry, 52,* 238–243.

Sobel, D. (1995). Rethinking medicine: Improving health outcomes with cost effective psychosocial interventions. *Psychosomatic Medicine, 57,* 234–244.

Sobel, D., & Ornstein, R. (1996). *The healthy mind, healthy body handbook.* Los Altos, CA: Drx.

Strosahl, K. (1994a). Entering the new frontier of managed mental health care: Gold mines and land mines. *Cognitive and Behavioral Practice, 1,* 5–23.

Strosahl, K. (1994b). New dimensions in behavioral health primary care integration. *HMO Practice, 8,* 176–179. (b)

Strosahl, K. (1996a). Confessions of a behavior therapist in primary care: The odyssey and the ecstasy. *Cognitive and Behavioral Practice, 3,* 1–28.

Strosahl, K. (1996b). Primary mental health care: A new paradigm for achieving health and behavioral health integration. *Behavioral Healthcare Tomorrow, 5,* 93–96.

Strosahl, K. (1997). Building primary care behavioral health systems that work: A compass and a horizon. In N. Cummings, J. Cummings, & J. Johnson (Eds.). *Behavioral health in primary care: A guide for clinical integration* (pp. 37–58). Madison, CT: Psychosocial Press.

Strosahl, K. (1998). Integrating behavioral health and primary care services: The primary mental health care model. In A. Blount (Ed.), *Integrative primary care* (pp. 139–166). New York: Norton.

Strosahl, K., & Johnson, P. (in press). Managing and preventing work disabilities: What every physician should know. *Strategic Medicine.*

Strosahl, K., & Sobel, D. (1996). Behavioral health and the medical cost offset effect: Current status, key concepts and future applications. *HMO Practice, 10,* 156–162.

VonKorff, M., Katon, W., Bush, T., Lin, E., Simon, G., Saunders, K., Ludman, E., Walker, E., & Unutzer, J. (in press). Treatment costs, cost offset and cost effectiveness of collaborative management of depression. *Psychosomatic Medicine.*

6

Training Psychologists in the Era of Managed Care

Hanna Levenson
Levenson Institute for Training
San Francisco

Joanna Burg
Northwestern University Medical School
Chicago

It is easier to move a cemetery than to change a college curriculum.
An academic wit, (cited in VanDyke and Schlesinger, 1997, p. 47)

Economic pressures are focusing [our] attention.
—R. E. Meyer (1997, p. 63)

There is no universal agreement within the profession as to the appropriate role of managed care in mental health care delivery.[1] Although most psychologists are participating to some extent as providers within managed care plans (Davidovitz & Levenson, 1995; Murphy, DeBernard, & Shoemaker, 1998), many view managed care as having a "dramatically negative" impact on psychological practice (Benedict & Phelps, 1998). Some advocate for the importance of making a place for psychology in the managed care market (Hoyt, 1995; Zimet, 1989). Others perceive that managed care is the polar opposite of

---

[1]Several knowledgeable individuals have observed that the current era of managed behavioral health is about to be replaced with other systems of health care. Although we refer throughout the chapter to managed health care as though it were a monolithic force, we realize that there are great differences among various plans and that alternative models are afoot. Nonetheless, we believe this chapter is still relevant, because no matter what the future of mental health care provision, we are not going back to the way things were and there are important training issues to be considered as we go forward.

quality of care, calling it "managed cost" because of the system's focus on the financial bottom line (Miller, 1996), and even "mangled care" because of the limited quantity and poor quality of service (Franko & Erb, 1998). Given the widespread professional involvement psychologists have with managed health care (MHC) combined with the equally widespread dissatisfaction with many aspects of MHC, it is crucial that psychologists be prepared to address the challenges of this rapidly changing health care market.

With this conflicted and confusing state of affairs among practicing clinicians, it is no wonder that there is absolutely no consensus about the relevance, importance, and/or necessity of training present and future psychologists to deal with the influence of managed care. With the exception of prescribing privileges, perhaps no other issue has so divided psychology and aroused more antipathy than psychologists' involvement with managed care.[2] Although both authors have horror stories to tell about their past experiences within MHC (one as a provider and one as a trainee), it is our viewpoint that ignoring managed care and wishing it would go away is not doing a service to our trainees, practitioners, patients, or the general public. Therefore we have written this chapter to help encourage critical thinking and about crucial and pivotal topics pertinent to training for future practice. Somewhere between an unexamined jumping on the bandwagon of managed care and a reflexive circling of the wagons around the status quo, practitioners and those responsible for psychological training need to examine thoughtfully and nondefensively what they are doing, what they need to do, and why they need to do it.

It is our hope that this chapter will be useful to graduate students (and perhaps even undergraduates) who are concerned about their academic training and future employability, to educators who are assessing or redesigning training programs, and to practitioners who are selecting continuing education courses and exploring ways to deal with the changing therapeutic and economic landscape. As Humphreys (1996) stated in his excellent article on the history and future of clinical psychology, "the best question is not how to maintain status quo, but how to use this crisis as an opportunity.... How can clinical psychology cope effectively with the change and continue to make a contribution to human welfare?" (p. 195).

Some of the questions we posit with regard to the impact of managed care on training are the following:

—Does training just need a tune-up or a major overhaul?

—Are our graduates in danger of being unemployable?

—How much should our training programs be driven by the present marketplace?

---

[2]The heat generated by even use of the term "managed care" is illustrated by a recent article in the *National Psychologist* ("use of managed care," 1998). Frank DePiano, editor of *Psychotherapy in Private Practice,* was reprimanded by the members of APA Division 42 because the publishers retitled the publication to *Psychotherapy in Practice and Managed Care.*

—Do we concentrate on the basics or specialization?

—If we train for MHC, do we become part of the problem rather than its solution?

In this chapter first we describe the past state of affairs relevant to training. Second, we consider the impact MHC has had on the field. Third, we present how attitudes and values are critical to any discussion of changes in training. Fourth, we describe several training programs that currently exist to prepare psychologists for practice in MHC. Finally, we review some recommendations for how trainees and trainers can grapple with the issues at hand.

PAST STATE OF AFFAIRS

For the first 65 years of psychology's history, psychologists were educated as scientists. Those who helped found the professional side of psychology came from other disciplines (Freud/physician; Pavlov/physiologist; James/physician). Peterson (1997) noted that:

> when psychologists entered professional careers, as they did in increasing numbers after World War I, they had to figure out what to do by trial and error, or if they were fortunate, as apprentices to a mentor who had walked the path before them. (p. 45)

After World War II, the climate changed dramatically as the country needed large numbers of therapists to deal with the multitude of psychiatric casualties returning from the battlefields. Through the Veterans Administration (VA, now the Bureau of Veterans Affairs) and the National Institute of Mental Health, the federal government funded programs in clinical and counseling psychology. Because of the involvement of federal funds, accreditation/accountability standards needed to be formulated and adopted. The basic outline for defining the goals and parameters for educating professional psychologists was put forth in the report of the Shakow Committee (American Psychological Association, 1947) and at a conference held in Boulder, Colorado (Raimy, 1950). The model of training adopted was that of the scientist–practitioner (the "Boulder model"), with the American Psychological Association (APA) responsible for the accreditation of academic departments. This process was originally designed for a system that had few, if any, third-party payers, and the original goal was to provide consistently high-quality applicants to internships at VA medical centers. For almost a quarter century, the scientist–practitioner model and the Boulder-style programs that emanated from it predominantly focused on training for academic research rather than training for practice. As recounted by Peterson (1997), at the APA convention in 1964, "impassioned practitioners seized microphones to shout that they had been betrayed by their professors. They had not been given the training they needed to meet the demands of professional life" (p. 81).

In 1973 the Vail conference on graduate education supported the appropriateness of a variety of educational settings and models. In the years following the Vail conference, students eager to get professional training in an atmosphere of abundant employment opportunities gave rise to the development of the Psy.D. and the formation of professional schools of psychology. In 1987 the report from the Conference on Graduate Education and Training in Psychology held at the University of Utah (sponsored by the APA) noted that there had been a proliferation of practitioner-oriented programs with a resultant rapid increase in the number of graduates.

At the Utah conference and at the National Conference on Internship Training in Psychology held in Gainesville, Florida, no mention was made of the present and potential impact of managed care on training at the graduate or internship level. In the Utah conference report, the point was raised that perhaps graduate departments should be responsible for the marketability of their graduates, but only because experimental psychologists, who had been trained for academic careers, were having difficulty finding academic positions.

Until relatively recently, most training programs focused on teaching long-term, individual psychotherapy to trainees planning to go into solo practice (VanDyke & Schlesinger, 1997). Those clients who could afford it received long-term, psychoanalytically based therapy, whereas very impaired patients received behavior modification. Third-party payers

> mystified by what goes on in the inner sanctum of psychotherapy, accepted the word of the practitioner.... Practitioners justified their treatment by quoting gurus, originally those such as Freud, Jung, and Adler, and more recently, to name only a few, Haley, Erickson, Goulding, Masterson ... (Cummings, 1995, p. 11)

IMPACT OF MANAGED MENTAL HEALTH CARE ON TRAINING

The impact of MHC on practice has been dramatic, but not all of the changes within mental health care delivery are a direct reflection of the influence of MHC. There has truly been a confluence of factors: consumers' interest in using psychological services and awareness of the interaction between physical and mental health, employers' knowledge about the impact of mental health on productivity, the rising costs of health care, an abundance of mental health practitioners, availability of third-party payers, demand for accountability, and empirical findings regarding treatment outcome, to name a few.

Nonetheless, with the advent of MHC, practitioners' beliefs and practices that had long been held sacrosanct were severely challenged. Slowly the impact has trickled down to the graduate and internship level. Whether for good or for bad, MHC has taxed the traditional identities of professional psychologists and therefore has influenced thinking about the training of current practitioners, as well as those of future generations. One major manifestation of the impact of MHC on clinical practice has been the resurgence of interest in brief therapies.

In order to assess the degree to which clinicians use brief therapy and their training in it, a nationwide survey of 4,000 psychiatrists, psychologists, and social workers was conducted (Davidovitz & Levenson, 1995). The findings for the psychologists reveal that almost 90% do therapy that is designed to be time limited and focused. In fact, 41% of all private therapy hours and 56% of all agency therapy hours were planned brief therapy. Psychologists reported significantly more clinical hours and a greater percentage of their practice devoted to brief therapy as compared to the psychiatrists and social workers. Psychologists also were more likely to prefer short-term therapy (33%), have a cognitive-behavioral orientation (23%), be a health maintenance organization (HMO) provider (48%), work in a group practice (23%), and provide services to a preferred provider organization (PPO) (59%). Another survey of independent practice patterns found that 84% of psychologists in APA's Division 42 (independent practice) were members of HMO or PPO panels (Murphy et al., 1998).

With regard to their training, the Davidovitz and Levenson survey indicated that half of the psychologists who were doing brief therapy reported that they had never had any course work in brief therapy. In an earlier survey of professional psychologists in California and Massachusetts, over one third reported having little or no training of any sort (even self-directed reading) (Levenson, Speed, & Budman, 1995). In the U.S. study, those who had received training rated supervision, consultation, and workshops as most helpful. Multiple regression analyses revealed that the amount of brief therapy training and the judged helpfulness of that training predicted self-reported skill in doing brief therapy, while age, years in practice, gender, and practice site were not significantly related. Although psychologists saw themselves as more skilled and experienced in brief therapy and preferred short-term interventions to a greater degree than their colleagues in psychiatry and social work, their training in this area seems to be deficient.

Given that a great deal of brief therapy is being conducted in the United States by practitioners who may not be adequately trained, a study by Evans and Levenson (1997) was designed to assess the degree to which training institutions are preparing future psychologists to fill the increasing need to practice time sensitive therapies. A questionnaire was sent to the training directors of all 165 APA-approved graduate schools and 370 internship programs. If training directors indicated that brief therapy training were provided at their institutions, they were asked to forward copies of a more extensive survey to the individuals directly responsible for teaching brief therapy. With an almost 90% response rate, 60% of the graduate school directors of training said their institutions had brief therapy training. Surprisingly the psychodynamic programs were more likely to offer brief therapy training than were the cognitive-behavioral programs. Eighty-five percent of those at professional schools claimed to have such training, compared to only 54% of the directors of academic programs. Of those teaching brief therapy, approximately half said they covered crisis intervention, and practice issues and managed care. With regard to educational methods used to teach brief therapy, surprisingly, the most common was role playing (52%), followed by audio- and videotaping of student cases. Manuals were used in approximately 40% of the trainings. The most difficult training issues based on the experiences of the brief therapy teachers were shifting paradigms, setting limited goals, adhering to a focus, and developing a therapeutic alliance. Again, surprisingly, the psychodynamically oriented courses were more likely to cover the topic of managed care as compared to the cognitive-behavioral courses (78% vs. 18%).

With regard to the APA-approved internships, almost all (96%) of the directors of training (with an 80% response rate) said that their internship setting offered brief therapy training. From these data, it appears that nearly all students who completed an APA internship have received some form of brief therapy training. Forty percent of instructors of brief therapy practica said their training covered practice issues and managed care. The most problematic training issues cited by the internship educators were setting of limited goals, attitudinal bias toward long-term therapy, and selection criteria.

In summary, although there is a high prevalence of brief therapy training both at graduate schools and in internship settings, over 40% of graduate schools do not expose their students to brief therapy courses or seminars. When it is offered, a high percentage of students take brief therapy training, indicating student interest and motivation. Despite the recent upsurge in the interest and number of brief therapy training manuals, only 42% of the brief trainings in graduate programs and 20% in internships use them. Nearly one half of the difficult training issues identified by educators come under the category of attitudes and values regarding the nature of therapy and the process of change (e.g., attitudinal bias of therapists toward long-term therapy, shifting paradigms).

Although Belar (1989) indicated that brief therapy was the model treatment delivered within HMOs, current practice suggests that HMOs often prefer a crisis intervention model or medically necessary treatment. She recommends specific training in what has been increasingly called "HMO therapy" as necessary for practice within managed care settings (Cummings, 1996).

According to a recent article on practitioner's perceptions of managed care (Phelps, Eisman, & Kohout, 1998), new graduates responding to APA's most recent doctorate employment survey (Wicherski & Kohout, 1997) said that they needed training to help them deal with the present realities of health care delivery systems. Austad, Morgan, and Holstein (1992) concluded, based on their survey of mental health practitioners, that current graduate education has not demarcated necessary skills and competencies for MHC practice. Seventy-five percent of their respondents indicated that gradate school training did not prepare them for work in an HMO, and almost two thirds said they had little or no knowledge of managed care. An expanded survey (Austad, Sherman, & Holstein, 1993) replicated these dismal findings, and the authors observed that practitioners "often struggle with the incongruences between traditional training and the clinical realities seen in managed care systems" (p. 12).

Hoyt (1992) commented that "most graduate schools don't do much to train people in the skills necessary to make it in the real world of clinical practice" (p. 80). Cummings (1995) chastised graduate schools for "training excellent practitioners for the 1980's" (p. 14) and predicted that only 50% of them will make it into the new millennium. Broskowski (1995) cogently argued that "one cannot reasonably discuss the future training and career paths of psychologists without considering the future of mental health care delivery and financing mechanisms in this country" (p. 156). However, he also concluded that his "own experience and history suggest that graduate education will follow, not lead, psychologists into the future" (p. 161).

With regard to the impact of managed care on established professionals' training, one has only to count the number of brochures that show up in mailboxes offering workshops on time-effective, solution-focused, or brief therapy. An abundance of books are also being published on the topic of short-term therapy (e.g., *Time-limited dynamic psychotherapy: A guide to clinical practice*) or business practices (e.g., *The essential guide to group practice in mental health*). Clearly many practicing psychologists are feeling the need to bootstrap themselves into more cost-efficient therapies and modes of service delivery. In 1997, *Psychotherapy Finances* surveyed its readership. Responses indicated that there has been a continuing increase in the number of therapists who are taking training in time-limited therapy techniques and in the number who say that they have adopted these techniques in their practices during the past year. Almost 60% of the psychologists reported attending a training in time-limited therapy in the past three years. (It should also be pointed out that master's level counselors attended such trainings at an even higher rate.) "Both the stampede into group practices and the rush to acquire new therapy skills are grass-roots phenomena by psychologists who are in the trenches" (Cummings, 1995, p. 11).

The influence of managed care on continuing education can also be observed in a backlash movement to train clinicians on how to survive professionally and financially without dealing with managed care. Recently, there have been a spate of flyers promoting workshops on finding niches in mental health care services (e.g., custody mediation for the courts, stress management procedures) where the impact of managed care has not spread, and a growing number of books and articles describing how to "break free" of the influence of managed care and "regain control" of one's practice (e.g., Ackley, 1997).

Although therapists in private practice are under increasing pressure to become involved in organized systems of care, over half of the respondents to a recent survey of 47,000 practitioner members of APA (Phelps et al., 1998) said they were spending approximately 75% of their time providing traditional services within an independent practice setting. Surprisingly, the survey also indicated that recent graduates are more likely to work in a private practice setting than any other place. Phelps et al. (1995) similarly found that approximately half of their sample was in full-time independent practice, with an additional third in part-time private practice. Murphy et al. (1998) in surveying members of APA's Division 42 (independent practice) found that, in general, respondents had not significantly changed their practice patterns, despite a reduced level of income for work performed. However, another survey (Saeman, 1996) found that psychologists over age 50 were considering early retirement; young psychologists were seeking salaried employment, and those in between were working harder and longer to maintain their incomes.

Whereas opportunities for professionals to gain further training exist to varying degrees in the private sector, within traditional training programs there is much resistance to including training modules on managed care. As Troy and Shueman (1996) note,

> One cannot be particularly sanguine about the likelihood of self-initiated and self-directed change on the part of training programs. The necessary contingencies are simply not there in the traditional academic world. One might hope that certain obvious moral imperatives might become a motive force powerful enough to energize programs into confronting the challenges of redesign. This remains to be seen, however. (p. 78)

Psychiatrists VanDyke and Schlesinger (1997) voice a similar viewpoint stating that in academia, "most change attempts arise out of belated awareness that what is being taught no longer corresponds to current needs or knowledge.... When the changes come suddenly and seem to require sharp departure from previous practice, the faculty may not be equipped by background, level and nature of skills, or by inclination, to present the new material competently and to serve as teachers, trainers and mentors for the next generations of students" (p. 47).

This perspective is supported by data. Resnick (1997), in a survey of accredited doctoral training programs in psychology, found that although almost 90% teach short term, problem-focused therapy, fewer than one third of the programs offer training in organized health care and fewer than 40% of the faculty have actual experience practicing within organized care systems. These findings indicate that most of the faculty do not have personal professional knowledge of managed care systems. Resnick also found that more than half of the graduate programs reported that they had no one on the faculty with expertise in managed care. Resnick concluded that graduate schools "continue to train people to do traditional one-on-one long-term psychotherapy despite the fact that the market for this type of care is dwindling, perhaps in the hope that they can get more and more of less and less " (p.68).

However, it is not just academia that has failed to accommodate the rapid changes now taking place. Few of the managed care institutions themselves have supported or undertaken training programs for their own staff or for graduate school trainees (Donovan, Steinberg, & Sabin, 1994). Budman and Armstrong (1992) found that few HMOs or employment assistance programs (EAPs) have a structured, planned brief therapy training program in place for their staff and/or trainees. They comment that there are administrative and clinical resistances to instituting brief therapy training.

In addition to the direct impact of managed care on training practices, its indirect effects have even more repercussions. Many anticipate that there will be an oversupply of Ph.D.s (Cummings, 1996) due to the fact that managed care prefers hiring nondoctoral level providers (Murphy et al., 1998). Internships have been particularly affected. Because most managed care contracts allow only licensed clinicians to provide service, many psychology predoctoral interns cannot be reimbursed for their work because they are unlicensed (de Groot, 1994). According to a survey by Constantine and Gloria (1998), 40% of internship training directors perceived that managed health care already had or would affect their ability to fund present internship slots. Almost 30% of the directors also indicated that their intern selection criteria were influenced by applicants' previous training in brief therapy and/or in managed health care. Some said they now had a preference for licensed interns. Furthermore, it has become increasingly more difficult for interns to find internship or postdoctoral positions, because these opportunities are diminishing as staff positions are eliminated. A recent commentary in the *APA Monitor* (Murray, 1998a) noted that due to budget cuts in the state of New York, a record 40 doctoral students were without internships. Especially vulnerable are internships in hospitals due to both the contraction of inpatient care and diminishing funding sources.

With regard to professional organizations' reactions to managed care, the response of APA initially was "curiously aloof" (Cummings, 1995, p. 11) during the beginning of managed care's inroads. Since that time, APA has spearheaded or collaborated on several training committees, task forces, and a demonstration project, which in part can be seen as influenced (if not caused) by concerns about managed care. For example, APA's Council of Representatives in 1995 voted to support the development of a new curriculum to prepare psychologists to prescribe medications, and the Department of Defense sponsored the psychopharmacology demonstration project. In 1997 the APA Education Directorate and Research Office, as part of a contract awarded by the federal government's Center for Mental Health Services (CMHS), appointed a "working group" to report on the implications of changes in the health care delivery system for the training and continuing professional education of psychologists. Division 12 (clinical psychology) designated a task force on the promotion and dissemination of psychological procedures (American Psychological Association, 1993), which devised criteria by which to define empirically supported treatments, surveyed the state of training at the predoctoral level, and put forth recommendations for the development of and training in such treatment modalities (American Psychological Association, 1995).

EMPIRICALLY SUPPORTED TREATMENTS

The need for psychologists to provide and promote treatments that have demonstrated efficacy has become increasingly important with the pressures of competing treatment modalities (e.g. psychopharmacology) and of managed care organizations. Data-based interventions are more readily defensible than treatments without clear empirical support, and consequently APA has become interested and involved in informing the business sector and the public about the availability of such treatments. Adequate training in empirically supported treatments (ESTs) at the predoctoral and postdoctoral levels appears to flow naturally from the scientist-practitioner model of training. Such training is critical to making ESTs available for public consumption.

In 1993, the Division 12 task force report put forth a list with examples of "empirically validated treatments" and "probably efficacious treatments" based on criteria they had developed. The list of validated treatments included 16 behavioral and cognitive-behavioral treatments for disorders such as depression, anxiety, and chronic pain. It also included interpersonal therapy for bulimia and depression, as well as a family education program for schizophrenia. The "probably efficacious" list included treatments such as brief dynamic psychotherapies, dialectical behavior therapy, and habit reversal and control techniques.

Results of a survey of directors of clinical training (Crits-Christoph, Frank, Chambless, Brody, & Karp, 1995) to assess the status of training in ESTs at the graduate level indicate that the average graduate program provided didactic instruction on 46% of the 25 treatments considered to be well established or probably efficacious. However, this figure may be misleading, as the range was 0–96% and no median statistic was provided. Forty-four percent of these treatments were reported to be taught in a practicum setting, again with considerable variability with a range of 0–92%. In addition, the extent of training by program was not quantified in the study. The report also found that over one fifth of programs offered didactic exposure to fewer than 25% of the so-called validated treatments. Overall, it appears that most graduate programs provide some introduction to ESTs; however, the extent of training has not been sufficiently quantified.[3]

The list of empirically supported treatments highlights at least two significant and related dilemmas in the field. First, although considerable research has been done in the area of psychodynamic treatment, behavioral and cognitive-behavioral therapies are more amenable to manualized treatments and controlled trials than psychodynamic psychotherapy. However, psychodynamic treatments have wide clinical acceptance due to observed effectiveness in the field (Seligman, 1995), and these approaches continue to be widely taught and practiced (Evans & Levenson, 1997). The Division 12 task force (American Psychological Association, 1993) addressed this issue by stating that "training programs may elect to continue to teach the[se] treatments in addition to treatments with stronger empirical foundations. In the long term, however, programs should increasingly move towards a concentration of effort in training students in those methods which rest on firm empirical support" (p.4).

The second dilemma raised by the EST movement relates to the value of highly controlled studies. Although controlled trials in psychotherapy research may be able to evaluate the efficacy of specific treatment protocols, there is

---

[3]Teachers and supervisors who are interested can request a sampling of graduate course syllabi being used for courses in empirically supported treatments. These have been complied by Division 12 (Division 12 Central Office, P.O. Box 1082, Niwot, CO 80544-1082).

concern that the data may not generalize well to real-world settings, where training is variable and clients' diagnostic presentations are often complex.

However, the spirit of endorsing and training practitioners in ESTs is commendable from many perspectives. The emphasis on ESTs is in keeping with the mission of the scientist–practitioner model to continuously evaluate practices. From a more practical position, psychologists need to be able to demonstrate that they are highly trained in ESTs to be attractive to managed care organizations. The Division 12 task force's recommendation that training occur not only through didactic exposure, but also through intensive supervision and clinical experience, fits well with the familiar apprenticeship model of training. In addition, the task force recommended that "APA enforce its current guidelines requiring documentation of the efficacy of new treatment procedures to be taught in workshops that are APA-approved for continuing education credit." (p. 8). In 1996, the APA's *Guidelines and principles for accreditation of programs in professional psychology* (American Psychological Association, 1996) mandated that training programs uphold the scientific basis of the profession by requiring that attention be paid to the empirical basis of therapeutic interventions.

The revised criteria require training programs to define their training models and philosophy, and support them with specific goals and objectives. Although specific models are not listed as acceptable or unacceptable, the importance of outcome measurement is emphasized. "There appears to be a new expectation that trainees be provided with a curriculum that prepares them for the opportunities that are available in the professional marketplace" (Shaw, 1997, p. 53).

However, it is unclear how responsive MCOs will really be to the empirical basis of treatments used. HMO therapy, or ultrabrief therapy, has come increasingly under attack by clinicians for lack of therapeutic utility and by researchers for lack of empirical data. Such therapy commonly comprises only 4 to 6 sessions, representing a shift away from the type of brief therapy practiced in the 1970s and 1980s, when brief therapy was defined as consisting of 10 to 25 sessions (Koss & Shiang, 1994). As pointed out by Levenson and Butler (1999), many of the models for short-term dynamic psychotherapy specify a treatment longer than that covered by managed care, which creates tension between what is being taught and what is mandated in practice. Most of the re-

---

[1]In a recent issue of *Professional Psychology*, an article titled "Innovative Brief Pithy Psychotherapy" appeared). The following are excerpts from that article: "Modern managed mental health care therapy, also known as pithy therapy, is expected to replace more traditional, lengthier forms of therapy by the year 2000.... Empirical studies indicate that providers find it therapeutic for themselves to provide it, and managed care organizations find it to be a cost-effective form of service delivery.... The focus of the therapy is to extinguish the patient's whining and to encourage behavioral change.... Those therapists who are proficient in one-sentence interventions will supervise other therapists, with the eventual goal of reducing an entire therapy session to three word, two, word, and finally one-word interventions.

search done to date has not focused on such ultrabrief therapies. As a result, ridicule of such HMO practices has worked its way into professional journals (Davenport & Wooley, 1997).[4]

ATTITUDINAL AND VALUE PARADIGM SHIFTS

For psychologists to succeed in the era of managed care, it will take more than merely learning a new set of intervention or business skills. Many therapists are reluctant to learn methods that have been shown to lead to better outcomes. Therapists' values and assumptions regarding the nature and practice of brief psychotherapy in general and MHC in particular contribute to this reluctance.

Budman and Gurman (1988) proposed that the value systems of the long-term therapist are different from those of the short-term therapist. These authors identified eight dominant values pertaining to the ideal manner in which long-term therapy is practiced and contrasted these with the corresponding ideal values pertinent to the practice of short-term therapy. For example, Budman and Gurman postulated that the long-term therapist seeks a change in basic character or "therapeutic perfectionism," whereas the short-term therapist does not believe in the notion of "cure" and prefers pragmatism, parsimony, and the least radical intervention.

Bolter, Levenson, and Alvarez (1990) sought to assess empirically whether, indeed, there were such value differences between short-term and long-term practicing therapists. Their study provides partial support for Budman and Gurman's proposal: Short-term therapists believe more strongly that psychological change occurs outside of therapy and that setting time limits intensifies the therapeutic work. Furthermore, results indicate that clinicians with a psychodynamic orientation, in contrast to those with a cognitive-behavioral orientation, are more likely to believe that therapy is necessary for change, that the focus of therapy should be on pathology, that therapy should be open ended, and that ambitious goals were desirable. Thus, although the findings from Bolter et al.'s study suggest that a short-term orientation is related to therapeutic values, it is important to note that the theoretical orientation of the therapist also plays a significant role in determining values.

Cummings (1995), influenced by Budman and Gurman's work, commented that for psychologists to succeed in the era of managed care, they need to make a "fundamental and pervasive" shift in values from those that are more traditional to those that are more time effective. He described seven of these paradigm shifts as follows:

(1) from few to many clients;

(2) from continuous to intermittent treatment;

(3) from cure to restoring drive to growth;

(4) from emphasis on the therapy to emphasis on the real world;

(5) from cure to as needed;

(6) from healing in the office to mobilizing the community;

(7) from fee-for-service to capitation.

The area of negative attitudes toward briefer modes of intervention is extremely important, because such beliefs could adversely affect therapists' willingness and ability to use brief-therapy methods effectively. Winokur and Dasberg (1983) wisely suggested that

> when teaching professionals a new approach, it is not enough to rely on lectures, reading materials, or even live demonstrations and individual supervision.... In order to integrate a new approach into their professional identity, particularly if this identity is molded already, they need to work through the intellectual, quasi-intellectual, and emotional difficulties encountered in the learning process. (p. 51)

Some data indicate that attitudes toward brief therapy can be changed with increased experience and training (Levenson & Bolter, 1988; Neff, Lambert, Lunnen, Budman, & Levenson, 1996). Levenson et al. (1995) found that for experienced therapists, one's attitudes toward brief therapy are predictive of skill in that area. Evans and Levenson (1997) found that teachers and supervisors of brief therapy in both graduate school and internship settings considered shifting paradigms and attitudinal bias toward long-term therapy to present difficult teaching issues. To the extent that present training programs promote values that are antithetical to brief therapies or MHC practice, future psychologists can be expected to be impeded in their effective use of such modalities.

TRAINING PSYCHOLOGISTS FOR MANAGED HEALTH CARE— SPECIFIC SUGGESTIONS

Educators who wish to modify the graduate school curriculum, internship experiences, or continuing professional education to be more MHC friendly run the gamut from suggesting a tune-up to undertaking a major overhaul. Some believe that psychology departments "merely need to tweak existing courses to include a market place focus" (Spruill, as quoted by Murray, 1998b, p. 30). Others (e.g., Troy & Shueman, 1996) perceive that "nothing less than wholesale redesign of doctoral training programs in professional psychology will suffice to meet the current and future imperatives of managed care and evolutionary health reform" (p. 58). Somewhere in between, Sabin (1991) states that "the skills required for successful HMO practice are continuous with already existing clinical skills.... When applied consistently in practice, however, this package of skills produces a unique product that is different from preexisting approaches to mental health treatment" (p. 608).

The push for change comes not only from educators and trainers. Wicherski and Kohout (1997) surveyed recent Ph.D. students, who responded that they wished they had additional training in business concepts, management skills, short-term interventions, marketing and selling oneself, understanding of and working with the emerging health care systems, understanding of the medical culture, and available roles and careers.

In preparing this chapter, we came across a variety of model curricula for professional training in the era of managed care. The question that immediately emerges for the educator or training director on seeing a list of such suggestions is, If these proposals were incorporated into present-day programs, when would there be time for clinical training? Educators are concerned that by focusing solely on such MHC content, case conceptualization, developmental understanding, and clinical skill may be undeveloped in trainees.

The first author recently had a startling and impacting realization of this while giving an introductory seminar on time-limited therapy to third-year psychiatry residents at a prestigious medical school. At the beginning of the first class, she gave clinical examples and research findings to suggest that briefer interventions could be helpful. Instead of the usual onslaught of resistance from trainees who had been indoctrinated in long-term therapy, she was faced with rather ho-hum acceptance. On inquiry, the students informed her that they had never done any type of therapy other than brief, focused therapy of approximately 10 sessions combined with psychopharmacological interventions!

In addition to recommendations for changes in specific content, educators have pointed out that it is not just skills and knowledge that must be taught, but also the manner and setting in which these skills are utilized. The need to learn how to work within a team and across disciplines is repeatedly underscored. Several authors have predicted that "the focus of our training will need to be changed because it is unlikely that professional psychologists in the future will be solely, or even primarily, direct service providers, the role that is most familiar today" (Spruill, Kohout, & Gehlmann, 1997, p. 7).

In vivo learning within a managed health care system has also been suggested as the best way to learn relevant skills and attitudes. As outlined by Charous and Carter (1996), training in such a setting is differentiated from traditional training by more of an emphasis on (a) the availability of a broad spectrum of interrelated services; (b) ongoing staff education in managed care policy issues; (c) supervision incorporating managed care concerns such as confidentiality, legal and ethical issues; (d) crisis intervention and management; (e) training in intensive documentation; (f) ongoing case review; (g) rapid assessment and initiation of treatment; (h) high level of therapist activity; and (i) judicious use of psychological testing.

In a similar vein, Sabin (1991) outlined six fundamental skills relevant to working in an HMO practice setting: (a) population-oriented practice management, (b) population-oriented program development, (c) application of an adult developmental model, (d) command of a broad repertoire of methodologies, (e) ethical analysis (sensitivity to multiple values), and (f) advocacy.

THE CENTER FOR MENTAL HEALTH SERVICES REPORT

The most comprehensive effort toward delineating the key components of MHC training was completed by the APA working group on the implications of changes in the health care delivery system (Spruill et al., 1997). This report does not constitute APA policy; rather it is a tool to help training directors enhance their programs. The report was prepared for the CMHS and is referred to by these initials in the following material. It included a comprehensive bibliography for various training areas that can aid educators in their development of course work. Although the recommendations are categorized by level of training (graduate, internship, postdoctoral, and continuing education), we summarize the main points more globally.

Clinical practice, supervision, experience with interdisciplinary teams, research, and course work were emphasized throughout the report. The concept of vertical training teams, in which students at different levels of training participate in the same training seminar and provide less experienced individuals with supervision and feedback, also was discussed. In fact, there was an emphasis on trainees learning how to supervise others as an important skill to acquire for practice in managed care organizations.

The CMHS report identified and made recommendations in eight areas that should be covered to adequately prepare psychologists for the era of managed care (see Table 6.1). Each is briefly presented.

New Systems

It is critical for psychologists to have some basic knowledge about MHC systems. For example, in the arena of health care financing, they need information

TABLE 6.1
Areas of Training Recommended by the CMHS Report

1. New and evolving health care delivery systems

2. Ethical issues

3. Multidisciplinary culture/knowledge

4. Clinical skills

5. Research

6. Business information

7. Technology

8. Health care policy making

on how to work with third-party payers, risks involved in shifting contracts, and discounting fees. Psychologists should also be informed about utilization review procedures, contract provisions, frequently encountered ethical dilemmas, and quality control. The CMHS report suggested that this knowledge base can be acquired throughout one's training through course work, professional seminars, continuing education courses, and finally practical experience working in an MCO.

Ethical Issues

Forty-eight percent of psychologists working with managed care reported ethical dilemmas created by the managed care environment (Phelps et al., 1998). The CMHS report identified several ethical issues that need to be addressed in training institutions. Working in a MCO raises issues of informed consent, abandonment (due to time-limited treatment), and confidentiality with regard to the third party payers and the use of technology that cannot provide a secure environment. Providers must also be aware of issues of competence, appropriate diagnoses, and divided loyalties. The report recommended, in addition to dealing with these issues through course work, developing peer consultation, joining the legal consultation plan offered by the National Register, and consulting with APA and state ethics committees.

Multidisciplinary Culture and Knowledge

Increasingly psychologists need to be prepared to work in multidisciplinary settings. Specifically, medical settings come with their own language, cultural norms, and political issues that need to be appreciated for providers to function effectively. Specific skill acquisition, such as behavioral techniques appropriate for patients with medical illnesses, is critical. In addition, whether or not providers ultimately work in a medical environment, it is likely that they will interact with primary care physicians and/or other health care professionals to provide comprehensive treatment.

Clinical Skills

Many of the specific clinical skills necessary for working in MCOs are already taught as part of the traditional curriculum. However, aspects of managed care present a unique approach to these skills. Providers should have a wide range of assessment and intervention skills available to them, and should be aware of how to choose the most effective path and how to communicate such a path through treatment planning to the MCO. Table 6.2 contains a list of some of these skills. The CMHS report suggested creating, in addition to courses and supervised experiences, a managed care environment within graduate training clinics when practical experience working in MCOs cannot be otherwise obtained. We suggest that even if other training can be obtained, allowing for such

TABLE 6.2
Skills for Managed Care as Outlined in the CMHS Report

1. Diagnostic and assessment

2. Clinical case management

3. Clinical and team supervision and teaching of others

4. Treatment interventions

a. Crisis intervention

b. Short-term interventions (individual and group)

c. Psychoeducational models of intervention, development of self-help materials

d. Long-term interventions (individual and group)

e. Some specialty service

5. Treatment planning

6. Research-based clinical decision making

7. Care of the seriously mentally/chronically ill

8. Quality improvement/utilization review

9. Specialty skills

training to occur within the clinic setting can provide the support and preparation to allow trainees to have more satisfying experiences once they are immersed in managed care. In addition, special attention should be paid to training in brief psychotherapy, including the attitudes, values, and skills necessary for providing effective and efficient care.

Research

Research skills are currently taught as a part of training in psychology. The CMHS report suggested a shift in the type of research taught and conducted. Psychologists are encouraged to emphasize applied research driven by clinical practice. It is important for psychologists to know how to perform effectiveness and prevention studies, and to learn how to market their services. They also need to be competent in technologies that are employed in both clinical and research domains. Trainees need training to become comfortable with information management systems that are frequently used by MCOs.

Business Information

Psychologists need to become competent in increasingly sophisticated management and business skills. These skills influence providers' financial, legal, and ethical well-being, and can impact providers' satisfaction with their practices. The CMHS report identified management and business skills to be targeted. For example, psychologists need to have skills in becoming an MCO provider, establishing a practice, marketing, and perhaps becoming a managed care administrator. The report stressed the importance of being able to understand fully the terms of agreements with MCOs, as well as the general health care market and how it might affect one's practice.

Technology

As technology is developed in the areas of information processing and communication, psychologists will need to be current in how these advances can be utilized in their own practices. Computers, CD-ROM, faxes, virtual reality, and the Internet are just a few of the available technologies that have direct application to the practice of psychology. The CMHS report suggested that broad-based computer literacy from word processing to scoring of assessment instruments be introduced at the graduate level. As psychologists advance in training they need to be aware of software for documentation, billing, and tracking patient progress.

Databases can be used not only for patient care, but also for archival research, literature searches, and continuous quality improvement. Technology may be directly involved in patient care, such as virtual reality desensitization training. Given the dizzying progress and rapid change in technology, "… psychologists will have to make a lifetime commitment to maintaining their technology skills and computer literacy" (Spruill et al., 1997, p. 73).

Health Care Policy

The final area covered by the CMHS report emphasized the importance of psychologists' becoming involved in mental health public policy issues in order to "maintain their current power, status, and influence in the health care system" (Spruill et al., 1997, p. 77). Graduate education in such fields as public health and political science are important, as is staying knowledgeable with regard to relevant national and local issues. As professionals, psychologists can join local state organizations and become active in lobbying.

PRESENT PROGRAMS THAT EMPHASIZE MANAGED HEALTH CARE TRAINING

It seems likely that the majority of psychologists today are learning the skills necessary for managed care through on-the-job experience rather than any formal preparation or training. Most psychologists know firsthand the difficulty of being asked to practice in a way that is frequently at odds with their attitudes, values, and competencies. We, as psychologists, are now in a position to anticipate the challenges of a managed care setting, and have the opportunity to prepare both new and experienced clinicians so that they can enter the workforce aware of, if not fully prepared for, the unique pressures they will face. Given the special skills that are needed to be effective and efficient it is not surprising that innovative approaches to training are currently being employed around the country at graduate, internship, postdoctoral, and professional levels. These programs range from familiarizing students with the types of demands that exist in the current market to teaching specific skills that may become the standard of care in the near future.

Graduate Training

Traditionally, clinical programs have required their students to gain experience in assessment and treatment through practica in clinical settings. Such training may occur in a variety of settings, from university-based training clinics to private hospitals. Currently, some programs are offering practica in managed care-dominated or -influenced settings (e.g., HMOs). In this way, students have the opportunity to experience managed care within an educational and supportive context. It is likely that most practicum settings expose students to managed care by virtue of its prevalence in today's marketplace. However, exposure alone does not constitute comprehensive, programmatic training. HMOs that offer training to graduate students include Kaiser Permanente and Michael Reese in Chicago (Donovan et al., & Sabin, 1994).

Frequently students are trained at clinics sponsored and run by the psychology department of a given university or professional school. Often, training clinics in graduate programs are able to offer sliding scale fees and long-term treatment limited only by the length of stay of the student clinician. These sites may be the only opportunity for students to learn longer term therapy during their graduate training and are valued in this respect. However, they can also be used creatively as a tool for training in managed care. For example, Colorado State University has developed a program for advanced graduate students that mimics a managed care setting as described by J.A. Kuhn (personal communication, March 10, 1998). Students take a didactic seminar on professional issues, including managed care practice. They select two clients from their case load of six to eight to be their managed care cases. During the initial stage of treatment they are asked to complete a two page form requesting additional services along with DSM-IV diagnoses. A specific and measurable treatment plan, as well as goals with behavioral indicators of progress toward those goals and the number and frequency of future sessions, is required. When the request form is completed, the clinic manager acts as the managed care company reviewer. Student therapists are typically given three additional sessions before they are required to complete their next request. Unlike a managed care company, the clinic manager also provides feedback on better ways to operationalize terms and to communicate such information to third-party payers. Although such programs may not replicate the real-world experience, they certainly allow for familiarization of the current managed care practices in a supportive and instructive setting.[5]

Internship Training

Internship year is currently framed as an intensive clinical training experience that occurs at the predoctoral level. It typically involves several specialty rotations as well as seminars and intensive supervision. Clearly, it is an optimal time for psychology students to be exposed to, and have formal training in, issues relevant to managed care. Several sites have developed creative training programs designed to train psychologists for the unique demands of managed care.

Charous and Carter (1996) reported on a training program that has been introduced in the Department of Psychiatry and Behavioral Medicine at the Medical College of Wisconsin. This training takes place in the department's behavioral medicine clinic, which contracts with managed care companies. Although the authors indicate that elements of traditional training exist in this setting, they describe several aspects that differ from conventional programs including ongoing staff education in managed care policy issues (such as determination of necessity for treatment and utilization review procedures) and supervision dealing with managed care concerns such as confidentiality, legal and ethical issues, and compromised professional autonomy. Introducing psy-

---

[5]One graduate program that is a product of managed care was developed by Michael Jospe, Ph.D. for the California School of Psychology Los Angeles (CSPPLA) (CSPP, 1998; M. Jospe, personal communication, Spring 1998). CSPPLA offers a Master of Behavioral Healthcare Management (MBHM) degree program targeted at training nonpsychologists to work in managed care settings. Students in this program are often managed care professionals seeking advanced training to better prepare themselves for the real world demands of managed care. They can specialize in case management, quality assurance/quality management, or provider operations and network management. Dr. Jospe emphasizes that this allows managed care professionals to be trained outside of managed care organizations, allowing for improved understanding of the training and practice of psychology, and potentially for productive partnerships between managed care and mental health professionals. He feels that this is a proactive approach that has the potential of increasing the influence of psychology on the practice of managed care.

CSPPLA is offering courses in at least five areas. There are courses such as diagnosis and treatment overview and case management and treatment planning. Courses in health care organization, provider operations, and network management are also offered, as well as courses in regulatory issues, and program evaluation and quality management. Finally, there are courses in finance, such as principles of behavioral health services financing and marketing, and principles of financial analysis. The advantage to having such a program in the context of a psychology program is that it allows psychology students to benefit from these courses as well.

chologists to these and other training issues in a multidisciplinary setting makes good sense in the context of increasing roles for psychologists in the area of behavioral medicine within the managed care framework.

The involvement of psychologists in the primary care setting has been identified as an important area for professional development in psychology as medicine becomes increasingly organized around primary care physicians. Zilberg and Carmody (1995) discussed the development of the Primary Care Education (PRIME) program at the Department of Veterans Affairs (VA) Medical Center in San Francisco in terms of the implications for training psychologists for managed care. The PRIME program is a VA initiative that calls for the development of comprehensive, interdisciplinary treatment of medical patients through which trainees prepare for the changing health care delivery system. This system redirects patients away from specialty treatment and toward utilizing their primary care providers as the pivot point for their treatment. The VA funded 24 sites for this program and allowed each site significant flexibility to determine the exact structure. Psychology was included in this funding, presenting an opportunity for internship training to expand into the area of primary care.

In the San Francisco VA PRIME program all interns are required to participate in a 6-month primary care rotation wherein they are housed in the same clinic as primary care residents and other trainees from a variety of disciplines. Interns accept referrals and provide consultation. Zilberg and Carmody (1995) commented that interns needed to have available a wide range of skills in order to meet the challenge of responding to the diverse patient population and treatment requests. They maintained that psychologists should preserve and develop an "in-depth generalist" model of training, particularly in the predoctoral stages, in order to be able to effectively deliver services and function as the "gate keepers" to more specialized mental health treatment.

The San Francisco VA Medical Center also houses a rotation for psychology interns and psychiatry residents in time-limited dynamic psychotherapy (TLDP). This program is directed by Hanna Levenson, Ph.D., and is of particular relevance not only because of its focus on brief training, but also because the structure of the program lends itself well to potential training in and for a managed care environment. Approximately five trainees participate in the 6-month rotation wherein they treat one or two cases with TLDP and videotape each session. Levenson meets with the trainees as a group weekly for 3 hours. The first hour is spent with didactics that address general topics in brief psychotherapy as well as issues that are relevant to the current stage of treatment (e.g., case formulation at the beginning, termination issues at the end). Levenson uses a variety of tools in her teaching such as a treatment manual, videotaped segments of her own clinical work, as well as that of previous trainees edited to illustrate various techniques and principles, and planned exercises (e.g., role playing). The second portion of the class is group supervision. Trainees videotape each therapy session and select a brief (5- to 10-minute) section of that week's session to present to the group. In this way, trainees have the opportunity to observe how TLDP applies to their individual cases, as well as how it is adapted to different patient–therapist dyads. Consequently, trainees are exposed to several cases in an intensive fashion in a time-efficient manner.

As part of this rotation, Levenson conducts research on brief therapy outcome (Bein, Levenson, & Overstreet, 1994) and the impact of training and supervision in brief therapy (Bolter et al., 1990; Levenson & Bolter, 1988; Levenson et al., 1995). This model of combining didactics, supervision, and research into a clinical training rotation provides an example of the multiple roles that psychologists need to fulfill within a managed care setting. Use of training settings as an opportunity for research not only demonstrates the implementation of the scientist-practitioner model for trainees, but also allows psychologists to respond to the need for establishing and documenting effective treatment and training interventions.

Postdoctoral Training

The Harvard Community Health Plan is an HMO that houses the largest and most established managed mental health care training program in the country (Donovan et al., 1994). It is a 12-month, half-time program that trains psychiatric residents, postdoctoral psychologists, nurses, and social workers at the post-master's degree level. Trainees have the opportunity to experience managed mental health care in the context of a well-developed training program. According to its founders, the program benefits both the trainees and the HMO. Trainees experience the challenges of managing a large caseload (with two new patients per week), along with learning how to develop comprehensive, focused, effective, and ethical treatment approaches. The HMO benefits by promoting academic endeavors such as training and research, as well as developing a well-trained pool of job applicants. The program's brochure states that in the past 14 years, 56 graduates have been hired to staff positions.

During the course of the 12-month program, trainees participate in a weekly seminar that meets for 2½ hours. This seminar serves as the organizing force of the training experience, providing phase specific didactics, support, and experiential exercises. The content areas that are covered include an introduction to managed care issues, evaluation, crisis intervention, individual brief treatment, short-term group, family and couple treatment, specialty approaches to treatment for specific disorders (e.g., PTSD and substance abuse), and termination. Clearly this is an ambitious agenda, and the trainers are concerned about issues of breadth versus depth.

In addition to the content of the seminar, Donovan and colleagues describe several group process exercises included to facilitate learning. One area that they address is "the crunch." This occurs when trainees find that they have more patients than time in a day and must make treatment decisions in order to manage their patient panels effectively. They conclude that this is one of the most affectively charged times of the training and can be viewed as an opportunity for significant learning when trainees are encouraged to discuss their reactions within the context of the seminar.

In summary, the Harvard Community Health Plan appears to be an ambitious training model for introducing advanced trainees to HMO managed mental health care. Donovan, Steinberg, and Sabin do describe, however, several ongoing challenges. First, there is a paucity of theoretical and empirically based literature on the effectiveness of treating a large number of new patients in a pressure situation. Second, there is also a lack of research regarding effective training methods in this setting. Third, there is a parallel process that appears to occur—How does one do justice to the complexity of the material within a limited time frame? However, given the potential limitations, this program has devised a training structure that has impacted not only the trainees who have completed the program, but also the literature regarding brief psychotherapy and effective means of training.

Continuing Education

Many practitioners today are facing managed care challenges without the benefit of formal training during their pre- or postdoctoral years. The lack of interest of the MCO to provide such training for its employees, observed by Budman and Armstrong at the close of the 1980s, still seems evident today. To fill this void, a small but growing number of agencies, individual educators, and professional schools are offering continuing education courses, workshops, and certification programs in the areas of clinical theory and intervention, business skills, and administration relevant to MHC. The quality of these educational opportunities is variable. Other than APA-approved continuing education courses and the like, there has not been a built-in quality control mechanism to oversee or evaluate such programs, and the individual practitioner usually has only the reputation of the presenter or institution to go by.

RECOMMENDATIONS

1. The polemics involved in dealing with MHC vis à vis training have become so extreme that valuable perspectives have been lost. We hope training institutions can use MHC pressures as a wake up call rather than as a death knell or a call to arms.
2   We feel strongly that those individuals involved in clinical education (administrators, teachers, students) should use the particular juncture between managed care and training as a platform for a much needed dialogue. The tension between quality of care and cost of service must be addressed at the teaching level. To teach as though the whirlwind of managed health care were not a reality is a travesty; conversely, to let political pressures and market forces determine what and how future and present practitioners are taught will undermine completely a field built on clinical and empirical integrity. Graduate schools, internship settings, and continued education programs need to assist trainees in figuring out how to deal with complicated situations that constantly emerge in the MHC environment by balancing

clinically sound, empirically supported, and ethical decision making with resource (e.g., time, energy, money) considerations.

A good starting place for individuals involved with training to prepare for such a dialogue is the CMHS report (i.e., *Final Report of the American Psychological Association Working Group on the Implications of Changes in the Health Care Delivery System for the Education, Training and Continuing Professional Education of Psychologists* (Spruill et al., 1997)). This thoughtful and thorough report can be obtained through APA by calling (202) 336-5980.

3. Regardless of present market forces, we, as psychologists, must not lose sight of the fact that most of us chose our profession in order to be of help to patients. It appears from current surveys that many practitioners are prepared to reduce their income markedly rather than adopt practices that they believe are not conducive to behavioral change or amelioration of suffering. Although there is a substantial and growing empirical literature that indicates psychologists can be of great help to patients by using time-efficient techniques embedded in the context of a good working relationship, data regarding the efficacy of ultrabrief interventions delivered as disembodied techniques without regard to the interpersonal context are nonexistent or unsupported. All relevant empirical findings need to be communicated to both practitioners and MHC entities in a manner they are more likely to hear and appreciate.

4. As psychologists we must be vigilant that we do not convince ourselves that what is required in a particular situation is necessarily best. We obviously need to teach students how to prioritize and deliver care in contexts of diminished resources and/or overwhelming demands. However, we must be cautious not to glorify such make-do interventions or high-pressure situations (e.g., the crunch).[6]

5. The major question for those involved with training is how much the content of the curriculum should be steered by MHC forces. How does one weigh therapy versus nontherapy requirements? It is our opinion that clinical training should not be driven by MHC needs. First, as recent surveys indicate, many psychologists continue to practice more or less as usual despite the MHC environment. Second, there is no consensus that MHC is a desirable direction for our field. Third, this is a rapidly changing field. Nevertheless, trainees need

---

[6]In a personal communication, Michael Hoyt, a psychologist who for decades has been involved in MHC practice, teaching, and research, distinguished between present-day MHC practice and that of the past. In the past, he stated, practitioners knew they were trying to do the best they could with what they had, while recognizing that what they could give was sometimes inadequate. Those psychologists knew they were dealing with clinical and ethical dilemmas. However, he sees that the psychologist of today seems to practice as though the present shortages are ultimately for the good—leaving the practitioner operating in a more conflict-free (and, therefore, more dangerous) space. (For a cogent discussion of future trends and attendant ethical concerns regarding managed mental health care, see Hoyt, in press.)

skills that allow them to survive economically. It is our opinion that training for the predoctoral student should focus on the basics of skill development in observation, evaluation, formulation, and intervention. However, at the exposure level, beginning trainees should be informed about the changing nature of health care delivery and how this impacts the ways their skills might be utilized. At the practicum and internship level students should have opportunities to begin to deal with issues critical to MHC practice with appropriate supervision (e.g., case management, confidentiality, functioning within a multidisciplinary team). At the postdoctoral level more specific adjunctive training at both the informational and skill level can be added (e.g., business and management courses, nontraditional employment opportunities, use of technology, etc.).

6. Traditional clinical training methods need to be revised. Clinical courses and supervision are all too often unfocused. Training methods that more readily promote competency and skill need to be developed (e.g., use of videotapes in supervision and didactics, more directive feedback, opportunities for watching supervisors at work). For additional specifics with regard to training in brief dynamic psychotherapy, see Levenson and Strupp (1999).

7. Related to the previous point, empirical research on training is needed in order to learn which didactic methods work; training materials based on these empirical findings need to be developed.

8. The teaching of empirically supported interventions and conditions should be encouraged at the graduate, internship, and professional levels—but not solely defined in terms of specific treatments for specific symptoms (the so-called "empirically validated treatments"). What is preferable is focused training in a variety of well-researched clinical processes and procedures that have been shown to foster positive outcomes (e.g., therapeutic alliance, experiential learning) in both *efficiency* and *effectiveness* studies. As pointed out by Beutler, Kin, Davison, Karno, and Fisher (1996), it may be the managed health care movement that finally pushes researchers and practitioners to communicate with one another. Thus, we see the current trend of downplaying research in clinical training programs to be counter to the present urgent call for accountability in the marketplace.

9. It would be helpful if there were a clearinghouse through which information about innovative programs and curricula, resources, training philosophies, and the like could be disseminated and shared, so that each graduate school or internship setting would not have to deal with these issues *de novo*. Use of technology such as e-mail and the Internet could facilitate such communication on a more informal and immediate basis. Interaction with colleagues from other programs could facilitate broader perspectives and piggybacking of efforts.

10. Through a specifically designated entity within APA, helpful information (e.g., needs assessment of practitioners, lists of relevant materials or readings) should be gathered, analyzed, and fed back to

various training institutions. In addition, this also could be the setting
for developing modules of help to educators who are rapidly trying to
inform themselves. To some extent this has already begun (e.g., the
CMHS report). APA is also in the most apropos position to call people together to work on important issues and to disseminate this information more formally.

REFERENCES

Ackley, Dana C. (1997). *Breaking free of managed care: A step-by-step guide to regaining control of your practice.* New York: Guilford.

American Psychological Association, Committee on Training in Clinical Psychology. (1947). Recommended graduate training program in clinical psychology. *American Psychologist, 2,* 539–558.

American Psychological Association, Division 12, Task Force on Promotion and Dissemination of Psychological Procedures. (1993). *A report to the division 12 board.* Washington, DC: Author

American Psychological Association, Division of Clinical Psychology, Task Force on Promotion and Dissemination of Psychological Procedures (1995). Training and dissemination of empirically validated psychological treatments: Report and recommendations. *The Clinical Psychologist,* 48(1), 3–23.

American Psychological Association (1996). *Guidelines and principles for accreditation of programs in professional psychology.* Washington, DC: Author.

Austad, C. S., Sherman, W. O., & Holstein, L. (1993). Psychotherapists in the HMO. *HMO Practice, 7,* 122–126.

Austad, C. S., Sherman, W. O., Morgan, T., & Holstein, L. (1992). The psychotherapist and the managed care setting. *Professional Psychology: Research and Practice, 23,* 329–332.

Bein, E., Levenson, H., & Overstreet, D. (1994, June). Outcome and follow-up data from the VAST project. In H. Levenson (Chair), *Outcome and follow-up data in brief dynamic therapy: Caveat emptor, caveat vendor.* Symposium conducted at the annual international meeting of the Society for Psychotherapy Research, York, England.

Belar, Cynthia D. (1989). Opportunities for psychologists in health maintenance organizations: Implications for graduate education and training. *Professional Psychology: Research & Practice,* 20(6), 390–394.

Benedict, J. G., & Phelps, R. (1998) Introduction: Psychology's view of managed care. *Professional Psychology: Research and Practice, 29,* 29–30.

Beutler, L. E., Kin, E. J., Davison, E., Karno, M., & Fisher, D. (1996). Research contributions to improving managed health care outcomes. *Psychotherapy, 33,* 197–206.

Bolter, K., Levenson, H., & Alvarez, W. (1990). Differences in values between short-term and long-term therapists. *Professional Psychology: Research and Practice, 4,* 285–290.

Broskowski, A. T. (1995). The evolution of health care: Implications for the training and careers of psychologists. *Professional Psychology: Research and Practice, 26,* 156–162.

Budman, S. H., & Armstrong, E. (1992). Training for managed care settings: How to make it happen. *Psychotherapy, 29,* 416–421.

Budman, S. H., & Gurman, A. S. (1988). *Theory and practice of brief psychotherapy.* New York: Guilford.

California School of Professional Psychology (1998). Web site: http://www.CSPP.edu.

Charous, M., & Carter, R. (1996). Mental health and managed care: Training for the 21st century. *Psychotherapy.* 33(4), 628–635.

Constantine, M. G., & Gloria, A.M (1998). The impact of managed health care on predoctoral internship sites: A national survey. *Professional Psychology: Research and Practice, 29,* 195–199.

Crits-Christoph, P., Frank, E., Chambless, D. L., Brody, C., & Karp, J. F. (1995). Training in empirically-validated treatments: What are clinical psychology students learning? *Professional Psychology: Research and Practice, 26,* 514–522.

Cummings, N. A. (1995). Impact of managed care on employment and training: A primer for survival. *Professional Psychology: Research and Practice, 26,* 10–15.

Cummings, N. A. (1996). The resocialization of behavioral healthcare practice. In N. A. Cummings, M. S. Pallak, & J. L. Cummings (Eds.), *Surviving the demise of solo practice: Mental health practitioners prospering in the era of managed care* (pp. 3–10). Madison, CT: Psychosocial Press.

Davenport, D. S., & Wooley, K. K. (1997). Innovative brief pithy psychotherapy: A contribution from corporate managed mental health care. *Professional Psychology: Research and Practice, 28*(2), 197–200.

Davidovitz, D., & Levenson, H. (1995, August). *A national survey of mental health professionals on brief therapy.* Paper presented at the meeting of the American Psychological Association, New York.

deGroot, G. (1994, July). HMOs will not reimburse for some interns' services. *APA Monitor,* p.63.

Donovan, J. M., Steinberg, S. M., & Sabin, J. E. (1994). Managed mental health care: An academic seminar. *Psychotherapy, 31*(1), 201–207.

Evans, S., & Levenson, H. (1997, August). Brief therapy training in APA-approved graduate programs and internships. Paper presented at the meeting of the American Psychological Association, Chicago.

Franko, D. L., & Erb, J. (1998). Managed care or mangled care? Treating eating disorders in the current healthcare climate. *Psychotherapy: Theory, Research & Practice, 35*(1), 43–53.

Hoyt, M. F. (1992). Discussion of the effects of managed care on mental health practice. *Psychotherapy in Private Practice, 12,* 79–83.

Hoyt, M. F.(1995). *Brief therapy and managed care: Readings for contemporary practice.* San Francisco: Jossey-Bass.

Hoyt, M. F. (in press). Likely future trends and attendant ethical concerns regarding managed mental health care. In M. F. Hoyt, *Some stories are better than others.* Philadelphia: Bruner/Mazel.

Humphreys, K. (1996). Clinical psychologists as psychotherapists: History, future and alternatives. *American Psychologist, 51*(3), 190–197.

Koss, M. P., & Shiang, J. (1994). Research on brief psychotherapy. In A. E. Bergin & S. L. Garfield (Eds.), *Handbook of psychotherapy and behavior change* (4th ed.), pp. 664–700. NY: Wiley.

Levenson, H., & Bolter, K. (1988, August). Short-term psychotherapy values and attitudes: Changes with training. In H. Levenson (Chair), *Issues in training and teaching brief therapy.* Symposium conducted at the convention of the American Psychological Association, Atlanta.

Levenson, H. & Butler, S. F. (1999). Brief individual psychotherapy. In R. E. Hales, S. C. Yudofsky, & J. A. Talbott (Eds), *The American Psychiatric Press textbook of psychiatry* (3rd ed.). Washington, DC: American Psychiatric Press.

Levenson, H., Speed, J., & Budman, S. (1995). Therapists' experience, training, and skill in brief therapy: A bicoastal survey. *American Journal of Psychotherapy, 49,* 95–117.

Levenson H., & Strupp, H. H. (1999). Recommendations for the future of training in brief dynamic psychotherapy. *Journal of Clinical Psychology, 55,* 385–391.

Miller, I. K. (1996). Managed care is harmful to outpatient mental health services: A call for accountability. *Professional Psychology: Research and Practice, 27,* 349–363.

Murphy, M. J., DeBernardo, C. R., & Shoemaker, W. E. (1998). Impact of managed care on independent practice and professional ethics: A survey of independent practitioners. *Professional Psychology: Research and Practice, 29*, 43–51.

Murray, B. (1998a, January) Psychology leaders seek to revamp education, training. *APA Monitor*, p. 28.

Murray B. (1998b, January) Psychology trainers urged to update their programs. *APA Monitor*, p. 30.

Neff, W. L., Lambert, M., Lunnen, K. M., Budman, S. H., & Levenson, H. (1996). Therapists' attitudes toward short-term therapy: Changes with training. *Employee Assistance Quarterly, 11*, 67–77.

Peterson, D. R. (1997). *Educating professional psychologists*. Washington, DC: American Psychological Association.

Phelps, R., Eisman, E. J., & Kohout, J. (1998). Psychological practice and managed care: Results of the CAPP practitioner survey. *Professional Psychology: Research and Practice, 29*, 31–36.

Psychotherapy Finances (1997). *23*, 7.

Raimy, V. C. (Ed.). (1950). *Training in clinical psychology*. Englewood Cliffs, NJ: Prentice Hall.

Sabin, J. (1991). Clinical skills for the 1990's: Six lessons from HMO practice. *Hospital and Community Psychiatry, 42*(6), 605–608.

Saeman, H. (1996, January/February). Psychologists frustrated with managed care, economic issues, but plan to 'hang tough' survey reveals. *National Psychologist, 5*(1), 1–2.

Seligman, M. E. P. (1995). The effectiveness of psychotherapy: The Consumer Reports Study, *American Psychologist, 50*, 965–974.

Shaw, D. B. (1997). Managed care's impact on graduate psychological training programs In J. Schuster, M. R. Lovell, & A. M. Trachta (Eds.), *Training behavioral healthcare professionals: Higher learning in the era of managed care*. San Francisco: Jossey–Bass.

Spruill, J., Kohout, J., & Gehlmann, S. (1997). Final report of the APA working group on the implications of changes in the health care delivery system for the education, training and continuing professional education of psychologists: Discussion of knowledge and skills and selected readings. (APA CMHS Contract No. 96 MO2052201D).

Troy, W. G., & Shueman, S. A. (1996). Program redesign for graduate training in professional psychology: The road to accountability in a changing professional world. In N. A. Cummings, M. S. Pallak, & J. L. Cummings (Eds.), *Surviving the demise of solo practice: Mental health practitioners prospering in the era of managed care* (pp. 55–80), Madison, CT: Psychosocial Press.

Use of "managed care" in journal title lands editor in trouble. (1998, May/June). *National Psychologist, 16*.

Van Dyke, C., & Schlesinger, H. (1997). Training the trainers. *Administration & Policy in Mental Health, 25*(1), 47–69.

Wicherski, M., & Kohout, J. (1997). *1995 doctorate employment survey*. Washington, DC: American Psychological Association.

Winokur, M., & Dasberg, H. (1983). Teaching and learning short-term dynamic psychotherapy. *Bulletin of the Menninger Clinic, 47*, 36–52.

Zilberg, N., & Carmody, T. (1995). New directions for the education of clinical psychologists: The primary care setting, the VA's PRIME program, and the in-depth generalist model. *Journal of Clinical Psychology in Medical Settings, 2*(1), 109–127.

Zimet, C. (1989). The mental health care revolution: Will psychology survive? *American Psychologist, 44*(4), 703–708.

7

A Psychologist's Proactive Guide to Managed Care: New Roles and Opportunities

Nicholas A. Cummings
Foundation for Behavioral Health and University of Nevada, Reno

The entire field of health care in the United States has changed dramatically since the initial, unheeded warnings to the profession that behavioral health care was about to industrialize and that practitioners should move rapidly and assertively to preempt leadership from the impending corporations that would otherwise own this new industry (Cummings, 1986; Cummings & Fernandez, 1985). The modest prediction that behavioral care "carve-outs" would eventually grow to encompass as many as 25 million lives was met by skepticism, if not scoffing, that this was at best fanciful, and at worst grandiose. These skeptics have been stunned into silence as the managed behavioral care industry now boasts 150 million covered lives. In the meantime, practitioners have lost much of their autonomy and a great deal of the control over health care decision making. This first decade of managed care (1985–1995) has been extensively chronicled from the psychological point of view (Cummings & Sayama, 1995) and from the psychiatric perspective (Joseph, 1997), and is not repeated here. Rather, this chapter focuses on events since 1995, examining what went right and what went wrong, and looking carefully at the trends that are defining the already unfolding second wave of the industrialization of behavioral health care, with an emphasis on the roles psychologists will play in accordance with the opportunities that will be available to them.

Make no mistake: although the profession is still reeling from the magnitude of change occurring in the first wave (1985–1995), the changes that are about to occur within the next decade will dwarf what has already occurred. Many practitioners are still whining about what the first wave has done to them. The astute practitioner will study and understand what has happened, with particular em-

141

phasis on the emerging new wave since 1995, and prepare to meet the challenges and to take advantage of opportunities as they unfold. For those still mired in the past, the next few years will be disastrous. Those who find themselves excited and challenged by the future are the 50% of practitioners who will survive and prosper well into the 21st Century. It is for them that this chapter is intended.

AN ASSESSMENT OF THE PRESENT

Who Are the Winners?

The undisputed winners in the first wave of the industrialization of health care are those who pay the bills: employers, insurers, the federal government (which is the largest purchaser of health care in the world), and ultimately the American taxpayer. In the early 1980s the inflationary spiral of health care was out of control at a figure two to three times that of the economy in general. For example, while Detroit was chafing under the competition of Japanese automobiles, it complained that the first $1,000 in the cost of manufacturing an American automobile was the cost of employee health care. When Congress enacted the concept of diagnosis-related groups (DRGs), the rate of inflation of medicine and surgery settled at 8% annually from a previously consistent figure of over 12%, while mental health and chemical dependency treatment, which was excluded from the DRGs because no one knew how to include them, skyrocketed to 16%.

Suddenly, and for the first time, MH/CD (mental health/chemical dependency care) was driving the inflationary spiral for all of health care. The government, at a loss for what legislation to write as a possible solution, essentially left the behavioral health problem solely to the private sector. The government ignored outmoded laws, such as those governing the corporate practice of medicine, and gave a green light to the managed behavioral health care industry. The companies that were formed in response came to be known as carve-outs, because they removed MH/CD from the existing health plans and went at risk for that portion of health care delivery.

What has been the result? In 1996 the inflationary rate of health care was tethered to a surprising 4.4%, the lowest since 1960, after steadily dropping for the previous 3 years ("Managed Care," 1998). The credit goes to managed care; the winner is the purchaser of health care.

Who Are the Losers?

The Psychiatric Hospital.   The most drastic and immediate impact was on hospitals. DRGs reduced bed occupancy by as much as 50% in many hospitals. Nonprofit hospitals used to reimbursement on a cost plus 15% basis either went bankrupt or were sold to proprietary interests. For a time these proprietary hospitals made up for the loss of medical and surgical revenues by converting empty beds to MH/CD services and huckstering them on television. MH/CD inpatient costs soared and adolescent hospitalization became a growth industry. This was only a temporary solution for the hospitals' plight, for soon the carve-outs began to tether the runaway psychiatric hospitalization. The standard 28-day detoxification was reduced to a fraction of that, psychiatric admissions and lengths of stay plummeted, and hospitalization for the simple problems of adolescence was no longer acceptable. The hospitals fought hard against the intrusions of behavioral managed care companies, but eventually they had to cooperate because it was a matter of less business versus no business. The carve-outs had simply gravitated to the more desperate, and thus more cooperative, hospitals to the exclusion of the recalcitrant ones.

To this day hospitals are only marginally viable economic entities, and the more progressive ones have added partial hospitalization and a host of other profit centers that are part of the continuum of care that managed care has made possible. Many have partnered with physicians to form a kind of managed care company of their own, the so-called "physician hospital organization." Some of these have been successful but most have not. The hospital has a difficult time making a paradigm shift from its age-old function of filling hospital beds, something that is incompatible with the growing trend toward ambulatory care wherever feasible, in medicine as well as in psychiatry.

The fact is that hospitals were never conceived as being profit centers, and they have always been subsidized by charitable contributions and government funds. This raises the matter of the recent indictments of Columbia/HCA, which has come under the scrutiny of the Department of Justice for overbilling and double billing. Until recently, these practices were standard in the hospital industry for decades. The government looked the other way when hospitals billed Medicare and Medicaid as much as $25 for administering a bedside aspirin, for example. It was tacitly a way of keeping an economically impossible hospital industry alive. The difference with Columbia/HCA is that this was intended for the former nonprofit hospital system, not for the current proprietary for-profit companies. It is yet a possibility that the top executives of Columbia/HCA may be convicted of criminal offenses because they allegedly did not acknowledge internally that the economic culture of the hospital industry had changed.

The Private Practitioner. The impact on privately practicing psychotherapists took somewhat longer to become apparent, but it was no less devastating. Psychologists, who had struggled for years and eventually became the beneficiaries of the remedicalization of psychiatry, are particularly unhappy. They had become the preeminent psychotherapy professionals, only to find that their practices were dwindling, and the new competition was with master's level practitioners rather than with psychiatrists who had essentially abandoned psychotherapy to the social workers. Accountability, treatment plans, goal-oriented therapy, and standardized protocols became minimum requirements, and value-based purchasing and medical necessity determined who was treated and how. Nonfocused, more open-ended and nondirective psychotherapies were no longer reimbursed, and protracted treatment and especially psychoanalysis were the greatest losers.

By 1997 the methods of paying practitioners had substantially reduced the incomes of privately practicing providers ("Newsline," 1997). These included fee-for-service that had been negotiated downward, case rates, and only some capitation inasmuch as most practitioners were not prepared to predict and control their costs, and therefore go at risk. As price pressure increased on the managed care companies, they passed the "squeeze" onto the practitioners, lowering rates several times during the latter part of the decade. Finally, reductions in rates seem to have leveled off, with some indications of stabilization ("Peeks and Valleys," 1997), but by this time any lower rate would have made it impossible for the psychotherapists to meet their own overhead. Some energetic providers could boast that their incomes had remained stable, but they had to see twice the number of patients to realize this.

Clearly, practitioners were the losers in income, but they also suffered an additional indignity. No longer were they the sole determiners of the treatment process, as who received treatment and for how long were now the prerogative of the case manager. Accountability, outcomes research, and other factors initiated by the managed care era demystified what had come to be called "psychobabble." The payers, having a greater understanding of the treatment process, were no longer reluctant to disagree with, and disregard, the recommendations of psychotherapists. Loss of the decision-making role is probably greater than loss of income in fomenting of practitioner unhappiness, inasmuch as this is at the heart of the autonomy of the profession. But like the hospitals, which no longer determine admissions and lengths of stay, psychotherapists no longer determine their own treatment process.

A RETROSPECTIVE

Although much went right during the first full decade of managed behavioral health care, the list of what went wrong is far more extensive. In order to assess their impact on the future it is important to briefly review these.

What Went Right?

The Tethering of the Inflationary Spiral.   This is undoubtedly managed behavioral care's greatest accomplishment, as the previous annual inflation rate of 16% not only was economically unacceptable, but was driving the general health care rate of 12%. As previously noted, the managed care system has lowered the rate to 4.4%, the lowest in 37 years ("Managed Care," 1998).

The Continuum of Care.   Managed behavioral care has resulted in the expansion of services as well as the substitution of services. The number of persons seeking services and the number of practitioners providing services both increased, but both psychiatric hospitalization and the private practice of psychotherapy declined. The continuum of care was expanded with increases in psychiatric rehabilitation, day treatment, consumer-run peer support, residential treatment, and crisis programs. These results are based on studies by the RAND Corporation, William A. Mercer, Institute of Medicine, Medstat Group, Harvard and Brandeis Universities, and the University of California, Berkeley (Ross, 1997).

Integration and Coordination of Care. In contrast to the nonsystem called private practice, managed care has provided a vehicle for the coordination of care for the first time. Despite initial advances, managed behavioral care has yet to coordinate mental illness and chemical dependency treatments, and is lagging behind in the integration of behavioral health in primary care.

Accountability. Managed care has ushered in the era of data-based treatment. Mechanisms are evolving, but they still have a long way to go. In the meantime treatment plans and goal-oriented psychotherapy have become standard. The stage has been set for the emergence of treatment guidelines and eventually standardized treatment protocols, all data based. Also, in the meantime providers must justify and document treatment plans, something that was unknown just a few years ago.

Value. It can be said that cost containment has removed most of the "fat" in the behavioral care system, and now purchasers are concentrating on quality. Changes in the next few years will see value purchasing, defined as shopping for price plus quality. It is on the dimension of value that the look-alike companies must differentiate themselves, and all of this must be documented for the purchaser. A recent cost comparison study by Foster Higgins addressed the relative value of different kinds of health plans (Sherer, 1997). The cost gap between fee-for-service and health maintenance organizations (HMOs) widened to 17.3% in 1996, revealing that traditional arrangements have done little or nothing to reduce costs, while HMO costs continue to decline annually by more than 2.2%. In that same year fee-for-service costs not surprisingly rose 2.4%. Second to HMOs were preferred provider organizations at 13.5% below fee-for-service costs, and point-of-service plans were only 7% less costly.

What Went Wrong?

Loss of Clinical Focus. Once practitioners forfeited their initial leadership in managed care, it was inevitable that the baton would pass to business interests (Cummings, 1986, 1988). It is not expected that business interests would appreciate and understand the clinical process, but it also does not follow that in its lack of knowledge the business leader reject the process. Perhaps because of the fierce hostility from practitioners, perhaps by sheer expediency, or probably by a combination of both, the industry disregarded the available techniques that contained cost through clinical effectiveness (Cummings, 1988; Cummings & Sayama, 1995) and relied instead on the "bean counters." Nonclinical judgments are arbitrary, and they not only resulted in a plethora of malpractice suits but, even worse, precipitated the anger of the consumer, who translated dissatisfaction into complaints to the press and the legislature. A series of *exposés* on tabloid television followed, and a larger number of bills were introduced in state legislatures and in the U.S. Congress. The industry is currently initiating damage control, which may include a one million dollar fund for public relations.

Price Pressure.   Requests for proposal have increased in sophistication, but despite the lofty language, the determining factors for granting a contract have been three: price, price, and price! There are now strong indications that this is beginning to change, but the damage has been done. The highly competitive atmosphere resulted in behavior reminiscent of the old-fashioned gas wars, and the companies began bidding below cost just to obtain market share. In such an environment quality suffers at best, and at worst some companies cynically bid without any intention of delivering the services required in the underbid contract. In the meantime, the industry began to feel the squeeze, and managed care organizations (MCOs) stocks declined (Pullham & Winslow, 1997; Sherrid, 1997). The behavioral managed care companies took the heat while the purchasers, who were determined to drive prices as low as possible, were the real culprits. Whereas the public was outraged, the companies were helpless, as they could not point the finger at the hand that fed them. The federal government, which is the largest payer of health care in the world, was ecstatic that health care price pressure helped balance the budget, and members of Congress smiled benevolently when constituents demanded federal controls on managed care. So far, legislative controls have resulted in minor, cosmetic changes, but politicians are now experiencing the ire of their constituents, and the Congress and the state legislatures may enact some tough laws in the near future. We may witness the Congress, which promoted managed care for years, and the White House, which made managed care the centerpiece of the Rodham-Clinton health proposal, suddenly become the champions of reform.

The Squeeze on Providers.   Hospitals and practitioners were beginning to accommodate to managed care when the industry decided to pass on the price pressure by squeezing the providers of care. This was a mistake of unprecedented proportion. Now outraged, the providers joined with angry consumers and a fierce coalition was formed. Perhaps it might be said that the industry had little choice as the competitive market ultimately encompasses everyone. Nonetheless, the disgruntled bear was transformed into a ferocious grizzly.

Competitive Paranoia.   There is often a fine line between healthy and unhealthy competition. Unfortunately, the fierce competitive market in managed behavioral care spawned the latter. The American Managed Behavioral

Health care Association (AMBHA), founded in 1992, has never achieved the strength and prestige commensurate with the size of the industry it represents. Members were distrustful of each other, each behaving as though it were guarding its own "black box." In actuality, there are no black boxes, as everyone is doing essentially the same thing. Member companies withdrew from AMBHA for questionable reasons, and there was the added difficulty of members of the AMBHA board sitting across from each other when their respective companies were suing each other.

It is difficult to conceive how, at a time when attacks on the industry required a united front, anything could have gone more wrong. This is illustrated by just one of many unfortunate examples. CMG, a large managed behavioral health care company, won the large restructured Montana state contract, and Value Behavioral Health, which came in second, promptly sued. While this was going on, Merit Behavioral Care, which came in third, made an end run and bought CMG, thus becoming the ultimate holder of the Montana business. In the same year, probably not connected to the Montana situation but reflective of the general distrust that exists in the industry, Merit withdrew from membership in AMBHA, seriously crippling that organization and placing its future in doubt. Finally, in 1998, and perhaps a bit too late, the managed care industry began mapping strategy and building a war chest to combat the growing resentment of many of its high-handed practices ("Managed Care," 1998). In addition, merger and acquisitions occurred unabated.

Opposition to Integration with Primary Care. The carve-in is the antithesis of the carve-out, and it is not surprising that an industry that has grown to encompass 150 million lives and is fighting for its survival opposes it. Carve-ins refer to integrated medical and mental health systems, whereas carve-outs refer to the specialty mental health care companies previously mentioned. In predicting the industrialization of behavioral health care, Cummings (1986) pointed out that insurers abandonment of mental health benefits because of their inordinate cost necessitated the carve-out which could ultimately save the benefit. He indicated that this would be necessary strategy for about 10 years, whereupon behavioral care would have to return to its rightful place in the total health delivery system. There are now indications that the integration of behavioral health into primary care is emerging as the second wave in the industrialization of health care (Cummings, Cummings, & Johnson, 1997). The managed behavioral care industry does not understand this concept and fears it. Therefore, despite lip service, it is dragging its feet and even opposes progress toward the goal of integration. The innovator of the past decade has become the impediment to the next decade.

ENTER THE DEAL MAKERS; EXIT THE CAREGIVERS

It is difficult to make money in health care delivery. This author, who helped found the mental health system of the prototype of the modern HMO, the Kaiser

Permanente Health plan, recalls it as a "penny industry" inasmuch as the question was consistently asked, "If we do this, how many pennies will it add to the premium?" It is still a penny industry, but now we ask how many pennies will it add to the cost per member per month? Where, then, did the large amounts of money that have been made come from? They did not come directly from the actual delivery of services, even though profitability is important, but from initial public offerings, acquisitions, mergers, and other financial structures that are unknown to the caregivers but that are the lifeblood of the deal makers. In the past few years health care has become the province of the deal maker.

In predicting the industrialization of health care, Cummings (1986) warned that as in all sectors that have industrialized before, there will be a period of consolidation in which successful companies buy up less successful ones, and acquisitions will be used to increase market share. He predicted that by the early 21st century there will be somewhere between 6 and 18 "megameds" that control the health industry. He could not have predicted, however, the frenzy that has characterized the past several years. The health industry, being business driven rather than clinically driven, joined the "merger mania" that was sweeping Wall Street (Valdmanis, 1998), and it now appears as though the final number will be closer to 6 than to 18. It did not matter that most of the players were not making very much money, and many were actually losing money. In fact, most financial analysts were dismayed by the tissue-paper thin margins of the HMO/managed care industry in the face of enormously high prices being paid on merger (Sherrid, 1997). The following case illustrates this point

By late 1997 three managed care companies controlled 52% of the market: Magellan with 31.6 million covered lives, Value with 24.4 million lives, and Merit with 21.9 million. Magellan had just acquired HAI, Green Spring, and Vista; Value Behavioral Health had been acquired by Columbia/HCA; and Merit had just bought CMG. Columbia/HCA was facing fraud indictments from the federal government and was wanting to sell Value for needed cash, possibly to pay hundreds of millions of dollars in potential fines. It was hoping that the two natural buyers, Magellan and Merit, would enter into a bidding war, thus inflating the purchase price. Instead, Magellan acquired Merit for $460 million plus the absorption of Merit's $300 million in debt. Thus, over three quarters of a billion dollars was paid despite the fact that after servicing its debt, Merit was showing a substantial loss. Internal problems at Magellan made this even more incredible. That company had been flush from the sale of its hospitals, and a substantial amount of its revenue was dependent on regular payments from these hospitals, many of which during and after the deal with Merit were in default. The deal makers at both Magellan and Merit received substantial monetary reward, while the stockholders voiced their displeasure in lowered Magellan stock prices. When all the dust had settled, one company controlled one third of the industry and two companies controlled more than half. This was the largest deal in behavioral health as of this writing, but a number of similar deals revealed even stranger scenarios. Table 7.1 lists the 10 largest behavioral health care companies and their enrollments (Drotos, 1997) as of

TABLE 7.1

MCO Organizational Enrollment, a Comparison of 1996 with 1997, and a Brief Chronology of the Events That Led to the Reshaping of the Managed Behavioral Health Care Industry (adapted from Drotos, 1997)

1996 MCO Enrollment in Millions		*1997 MCO Enrollment in Millions*	
Value Behavioral Health	24.23	Magellan Health Services	60.00
Human Affairs International	15.44	Value Behavioral Health	24.39
Merit Behavioral Care	15.27	United Behavioral Health	11.30
Green Springs Health Services	12.44	Managed Health Network	7.08
Foundation Health PsychCare	7.50	First Mental Health	6.00
U.S. Behavioral Health	6.24	MCC Behavioral Care	5.73
First Mental Health	6.21	Options Health Care	3.87
MCC Behavioral Care	5.17	Family Enterprises	3.50
United Behavioral Systems	4.52	American Psych Systems	3.50
Family Enterprises	3.20	FPM Behavioral Health	2.50
FHC Options	2.69		
FPM Behavioral Health	2.10		

A Sampling of the Events That Reshaped the Managed Behavioral Health Field

5/94   Value Behavioral Health purchases Burke–Taylor, on of the largest EAPs

3/95   Value Behavioral Health acquires Health Management Strategies

10/95   Kohlberg, Kravis, Roberts purchases Merit (formerly American Biodyne) from Merck; Charter acquires Mustard Seed and Vista, forming a new holding company called Magellan Health Services; Magellan acquires the majority investment in Green Springs

3/96   Foundation Health Corp. acquires Managed Health Network

4/96   Aetna Life & Casualty buys U.S. Healthcare

1/97   Value Health joins Columbia/HCA

continued on next page

149

2/97	United Healthcare's behavioral health subsidiaries for United Behavioral Health
8/97	Magellan purchases Human Affairs International
9/97	Merit Behavioral Care acquires CMG, American Psych Systems acquires Principal Behavioral Healthcare
10/27	Magellan acquires Merit Behavioral Care

this writing, along with a brief chronology of the deal making of the past 2 years. This degree of activity in health care is expected to continue as long as Wall Street is in the throes of merger mania, a phenomenon that could vanish as suddenly as did the junk bond deals of the 1980s. Somewhere in all of this, if we look intensely, we might find the patients and their caregivers.

THE IMPENDING ERA OF THE PRACTITIONER

Industrialization: An Evolution

As practitioners contemplate all of the foregoing, it is no wonder that they feel intimidated by managed care. They may be skeptical that the second wave of industrialization will bring favorable changes. Yet the changes that are about to occur in the next decade will be as profound as those of the previous decade that have left privately practicing psychologists stunned, angry, and impoverished. Once industrialization takes place, there is no going back, but it will evolve. The purchasers of health care, who have wrested control of health care economics from the provider, will never relinquish their control. For years they waited for the inevitable glut of practitioners to lower costs. Once there were too many practitioners, costs increased instead of diminishing because the providers controlled both supply and demand, so the economic forces of supply and demand could not function. As patients became scarce, physicians increased the number of procedures. The word in medical circles in recent years was that it is not the number of patients one sees that determines income, but the number of procedures performed. Similarly, psychologists, confronted with fewer patients, increased the length of therapy accordingly and invented a series of heretofore nonexistent syndromes that need therapy. Thus, as many as 60% of boys in any classroom were said to suffer from attention deficit/hyperactivity disorder, depression was redefined to include the normal "blues," post-traumatic stress disorder was extended to any vicissitude of living, and for a time borderline personalities were encouraged by some therapists to mimic multiple personality disorder.

Cyclops and the IDS

The giant MCOs are like Cyclops, as they see only through one business eye. The integrated delivery system (IDS), on the other hand, has the advantage of two eyes: business acumen and clinical integrity. Of the IDSs that are competing directly with the MCOs, most are succeeding because once they have learned to predict and control costs, they are able to go at risk with a clinically driven delivery system that knows quality, is less imperiled by malpractice suits, and is relieved of the substantial overhead that plagues the MCO in its role, which has become essentially that of an arbitrageur, or "middle man."

For the first time in history, health care is subject to the forces of supply and demand, and the practitioners who learn this will be successful in their competition with the MCOs. Before discussing the form and strategy of such practitioner owned integrated delivery systems, it is important that the psychologist realizes that MCOs are not invincible. This author learned that lesson early when he thought in the mid-1980s that Maxicare (an MCO) would certainly be one of the surviving giants into the 21st century. The overnight demise of Maxicare is a lesson learned and now replicated over and over. Four examples, representing four distinct types of MCOs, illustrate the fragile nature of the giant. All of the following met their difficulties in the fourth quarter of 1997.

Columbia/HCA, the largest health care company in the world, is reeling under federal charges of fraud, which included excessive charges and double billing. Fines may run into the hundreds of millions of dollars, and some former managers may face criminal sentences. Columbia/HCA appears to be desperate to sell its behavioral care subsidiary, Value, and it may have to sell some of its hospitals before this crisis is over.

Apogee, another health care company that was once the darling of Wall Street, had the wrong strategy of buying up group practices. Its stock pummeled, and those who traded their group practices for stock are worth only a fraction of the original sale price after waiting out the required restrictive period before the stock was salable.

Oxford, the most highly respected of HMOs, because of its quality and unprecedented patient and physician satisfaction, lost 50% of its stock price in 1 day when it was discovered that its management information system was inadequate and had overestimated the revenues, cash on hand, and physician reimbursement.

MedPartners, which grew with seemingly lightning speed as it acquired a series of successful medical group practices, is floundering. Mulliken, once heralded as the epitome of the physician equity model (which included psychologists as owners), had its research and plans toward the integration of behavioral health into primary care derailed when it was purchased by MedPartners.

The lesson is that these giant "mega-meds" can stumble because they lack the second eye of clinical focus and integrity, and like the Cyclops of Greek mythology, their death can be sudden and painful.

Whither the MCO/HMO?

It is important for the practitioners who have formed, or are about to form, their regional group practices, or IDSs, to know what the playing field will look like in the next few years. The following are key issues to consider.

Consolidation.   Mergers and acquisitions will continue, and as long as the financial markets are characterized by merger mania, the health care field will not be off limits to the deal makers. Public outcry is building, and in the future federal regulators may be more wary of deals that resemble the acquisition of Merit by Magellan which gave one company one third of the market. Fueled largely by tax free "stock swaps," merger mania will one day end as abruptly as did the gigantic junk bond deals of the 1980s. But consolidation is inevitable, and eventually the health care industry, as far as the payers are concerned, will be dominated by a few giants.

Regulation.   An industry that goes from virtually zero to 75% of the insured market in a little over a decade cannot escape government regulation for long. Much has been trampled in the stampede toward cost containment, and regulation will bring about reconsideration within the industry. Practitioners are at the boiling point, and consumers have been subjected to frequent exposes of abuses. The Congress and the state legislatures will begin to micromanage the industry, but managed care in its next evolutionary state will survive and flourish. However, regulation could be fairly extensive and costly.

Self-Regulation.   In an effort to prevent undue government regulation, the MCOs will rush into accreditation procedures that are costly but still fall short of real evaluation. The companies that do not rush to accreditation will be punished in the marketplace. This process will create a large revenue stream for the National Committee on Quality Assurance, the Joint Commission on Accreditation of Healthcare Organizations, and other self-anointed accrediting bodies, and will place an undue financial burden on the fledgling IDSs and small MCOs, which lack the resources of their giant competitors.

Price Increases.   The outside micromanagement of the benefit has resulted in higher health costs which the industry is merely passing on to the purchasers. Late 1998 and early 1999 are seeing the inflationary rate move up again after years of decline. Eventually some of these price increases will reflect the costs of higher quality and expanded benefits, but for now they represent the effects of regulatory meddling that has reintroduced some of the waste, duplication, and ineffectiveness that characterized the health field before managed care. Other significant features that are increasing prices are accreditation, outcomes and performance measures, and lawsuits. Finally, after years of low-balling (pricing products below cost so as to grab market share away from competitors), most of the MCOs are hoping to make up for some of their losses through industry-wide price increases.

Universal Health Care.   Government ownership of the health system is unlikely in the near term, and industrialization will continue, but in modified form. There will be much talk and even more symbolism, but a series of incremental moves toward universal health care may add up to substantial change. Many psychologists regard government-sponsored health care as the solution to their practice problems, but if and when this occurs, it will be too late to solve the current economic crisis in the private practice of psychotherapy.

Parity.   Progress toward parity of mental health with physical health will continue as more states pass laws and existing federal laws are expanded. More than any other event, it is the implementation of parity that practitioners hope will save their practices. Such narrow parochialism can only perpetuate the separation of medicine and behavioral health and could substantially delay integration. More likely, however, there will be practitioner disappointment because of the loopholes that will prevent full parity, or the probability that parity laws will drive even more of the health industry into managed care (Stoil, 1997). True parity will occur when behavioral health is fully integrated into primary care, ending the schism between mind and body dictated in medicine by the 17th-century French physician and philosopher René Descartes.

Outcomes.   Purchasers will require independent, nonbiased documentation of therapeutic effectiveness and quality. Instruments will be developed, and outside research entities will flourish. With an emphasis on cost containment that is now clinically driven, medical cost offset research will become the most important outcome measure.

Treatment Guidelines.   Data-based treatment guidelines are close to reality. There is a national consortium of public, private, and government sectors devoted to this effort. Unfortunately, the research contemplated and underway is myopic in that it is taking the easy way out. It is concentrating on behavioral variables that are easily quantifiable, and the more difficult task of quantifying psychodynamic, strategic, and systems techniques is being ignored.

The Shrinking Behavioral Health Dollar.   As costs in behavioral health care have been tethered, the savings in dollars has not translated into expanded benefits, increased access, and renewed quality (Ross, Covall, Graham & Coakley, 1998). Rather, the dollars simply disappear into the system, with the behavioral health portion of the total cost of health care shrinking from 9% in 1992 to 4.5% in 1997. Consumers have a greater say in health care in the present climate, and it will be they who must eventually protest and curtail this 50% reduction in the proportion of behavioral health expenditures to total health costs. Such shrinking of behavioral health dollars, if allowed to continue, will result in a disastrous, almost irreversible erosion of the behavioral health benefit.

ENTER THE PRACTITIONER: NEW OPPORTUNITIES AND CHANGE

The emergence of large, prestigious purchasing consortia has remarkably changed the playing field. Initially formed to give the small business the same purchasing clout as the large employer by pooling the prospective number of covered lives, these consortia have grown into important buyer/consumer coalitions that have been rapidly educating themselves as to value. For example, the Pacific Business Group which began in San Francisco only 5 years ago, now covers eight western states. Providers who form IDSs now have a choice: they can contract with the MCOs/HMOs or bypass these and contract directly with a purchasing consortium. National presence can be achieved through geographically distributed alliances, usually through joint ventures, with other IDSs. Integration in these regional group practices is of two types. The first is vertical integration, which creates a continuum of all facets of appropriate behavioral health care (including chemical dependency, rehabilitation, hospitalization and partial hospitalization, day care, all outpatient services, etc.) Such an IDS is gaining momentum at the present time. Horizontal integration, on the other hand, represents the next wave in the industrialization and is just getting started. It involves the integration of behavioral health into primary care, so such an IDS involves primary care physicians as well as health psychologists and other behavioral care practitioners.

The Clinically Driven Behavioral IDS

Ever since it was pointed out that practitioners could form regional group practices and contract directly with the new purchasing consortia (Cummings, 1995; Cummings, Pallak, & Cummings, 1996), a surprising number of such groups have been established and are flourishing (Jeffrey, 1998). Using self-review, these behavioral health practitioners have learned to predict and control their own costs. Several large groups severed their dependence on the MCOs/HMOs, went at risk on their own, and are basking in what has tongue-in-cheek been called "the revenge of the shrinks" (Jeffrey, 1998, p. B1, B6–B7). Concurrently, many state Medicaid programs have been restructured to shift the risk of behavioral care services from the benefits payers to the providers of care (Oss, 1997), thus accelerating the trend toward practitioner-owned IDSs. Other group practices have maintained their connections with the MCOs/HMOs, but are now at risk, do their own case management, and are enjoying a new sense of autonomy and financial reward.

Even AMBHA concedes there will be a proliferation of provider-owned IDSs (Ross, 1997). However, there are a number of characteristics that must be a part of such an IDS, and these have been delineated by Edley (1996) and

Weinstein and Edley (1997), who are representative of a growing number of consultants who help providers establish and manage IDSs.

Size. Accreditation and performance measures have become costly items, and the IDS must be of sufficient magnitude to support these, as well as the even more costly conditions which follow (Weinstein & Edley, 1997, p. 40).

Network Operations. There must be a full continuum of care, with multispecialty practitioners and geographic coverage. These practitioners must fulfill the standards set by the National Committee on Quality Assurance, and they must be multidisciplinary, providing specialty needs and services as well as diversionary and crisis programs.

Clinical Operations. The IDS must have well-developed criteria and protocols of care. It must provide training in time-effective therapy, defined as "efficient, effective interventions, not merely brief therapy". There must be internal utilization management, and documented clinical and cost effectiveness.

Quality Improvement. Patient satisfaction protocols must be accompanied by well-publicized complaint and grievance procedures. The IDS must have developed clinical outcomes mechanisms, as well as an oversight and audit process of key functions.

Management Information Systems. Systems must be capable of patient tracking, with reporting of such vital information as utilization, cost, and the like. In the relatively near future electronic patient records will be standard.

Performance Standards. Standards must include access to care, telephone efficiency, and both geographic and service availability.

Administrative Functions. All three of the following activities must be centralized: billing, contracting, and single point of access.

Risk. The IDS must have the ability to contract with alternative reimbursement mechanisms and possess financial flexibility and viability.

Many existing group practices that fall short of this ideal IDS model would be surprised that with consultation and help they could achieve the next step in viability. This is especially true of groups formed to service the public sector, and if they combine public sector experience with private sector structure. Unfortunately, there are always those group practices that, mired in the outmoded thinking that a group practice is a number of like-minded psychologists practicing under one roof and sharing expenses and referrals, will unsuccessfully attempt this complex conversion to an IDS on their own.

Integration of Behavioral Health and Primary Care

Recently, the federal government and several private sector health contractors (such as the Pacific Business Group) announced contract incentives designed to accelerate the integration of behavioral health with primary care. This is not surprising, inasmuch as the "fat" in behavioral health has been successfully wrung out of the system, while the costs of somatizing, as well as stress-related and lifestyle-related physical conditions, are enormous. Figure 7.1 dramatically illustrates that a 5 to 10% cost savings in behavioral health pales in comparison to a 5 to 10% savings in medicine and surgery. Medical cost offset research has demonstrated consistently over 30 years that such savings are to be expected with the introduction of behavioral care interventions into primary care (Cummings, 1997a), and the medical cost offset increases with the degree of behavioral and primary care integration. As is seen in Fig. 7.1, a 7% decrease

MH/CD   Med-Surg

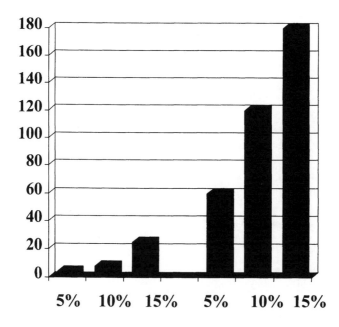

FIG. 7.1.   Reduction in billions of dollars potentially at the 5, 10, and 15% levels for the U.S. mental health/chemical dependency budget (first three columns) and these percentages for the nation's medical/surgical budget (last three columns).

in physical costs exceeds the entire MH/CD budget of the United States. A clinically driven, cost-conscious integrated system is the best way to address such adverse health costs in the future.

The integration of behavioral health with primary care has commanded much recent attention, most of which has been lip service. Few practitioners and health care managers fully comprehend the medical, social, and economic forces that mandate this next step in the evolution of health care. Equally confusing are the forces arrayed against this change, which range from the traditional manner in which care is dispensed to more recent innovations in health care delivery such as the carve-outs that are struggling to find their niche. The integration of behavioral health in primary care is in its infancy, and visionary providers will move swiftly to take advantage of the time lag.

Educational Process. Most psychologists fear that integration will result in loss of identity, whereas physicians fear the undermining of their authority and preeminence. Reeducation is a sensitive and painstaking process that cannot be hurried or forced. One must begin with psychologists who appreciate the importance of integration and who then will seek out physicians or physician groups that are aware of the pressure that behavioral health problems place on a health system and the physicians' harried schedules. One year of meeting, discussing, exchanging ideas and fears, examining the data, and eventually planning toward integration is an absolute minimum initial time investment.

The Physician Equity Model. In a fully integrated system it is important that both physicians and psychologists be eligible for participant ownership. This will assure that behavioral health and primary care are truly integrated with both sets of practitioners (primary care physicians and behavioral health specialists) appropriately involved in the decision-making process. The physician equity model has been extensively described elsewhere (Cummings, 1995, 1996) and is not repeated here.

Planning. This is uncharted waters, although there are a number of excellent examples of integration currently underway, at various stages of development. These have been assembled in one volume, and planners should thoroughly acquaint themselves with these efforts and even arrange on-site visits when possible (Cummings et al., 1997).

Financing. Capital acquisition for an IDS has been extensively discussed by Cummings (1996) and is not repeated here. However, a relevant issue is the matter of buy-in by the participating practitioners. Physicians are used to investing tens of thousands of dollars of their individual monies when forming a group practice, and psychologists accustomed to getting by with a desk and a couple of therapy chairs will find this degree of commitment foreign and frightening. A reexamination of this outmoded attitude may be necessary (Cummings, 1997b).

Management. The health landscape is cluttered with the carcasses of practitioner groups that failed because management was not authorized to make decisions but rather had to wait for the group to act as a whole. The number of such casualties makes it imperative that management is empowered to manage, and because both physicians and psychologists often attach an inflated degree of importance to their own management ability, it may be wise to retain a management services organization.

Degree of Integration. The integration of behavioral health in primary care is not an all-or-none affair. Rather, there is a continuum in the degree of integration from the very simple 1-800 number by which a primary care physician (PCP) can seek the consultation of a behavioral health specialist (BHS), usually a health psychologist or a psychiatric nurse practitioner, 24 hours a day. Population- and disease-based teams of BHSs and PCPs—with the obliteration of the traditional departments of medicine, psychiatry, pediatrics, and so forth— represent the ultimate in integration. Examples are pain clinics, back clinics, teen-age clinics, and many others (see Cummings, Cummings & Johnson, 1997, for an extensive listing and description) where each of these has its own budget, treatment personnel, and support staff. The midpoint between these two extremes of integration, as illustrated in Fig. 7.2, involves having a BHS on site, an arrangement that shows a significant increase in both collaboration and medical cost offset.

Disease- and Population-Based Protocols and Treatment Teams. Most psychologists have not been trained in the concept of disease- and population-based treatment programs that involve teams of PCPs and BHSs. This has proven particularly efficacious in chronic conditions ranging from depression and borderline personality disorder to the management of rheumatoid arthritis and diabetes (see Cummings et al., 1997, for an extensive list and description). Most behavioral health practitioners require not only additional training in health psychology, but also some extensive reordering of their roles.

Therapy Referral Compliance. A well-known fact is that only 10% of those referred for psychotherapy by a PCP ever follow through (Ackley, 1997). However, in an integrated system where a BHS is on site and the PCP walks the patient down the hall and introduces the patient to the psychologist, the follow through by the patient with a treatment plan is a startling 80% (Cummings et al., 1997).

It is difficult to predict the rapidity of the integration of behavioral health into primary care, as need and interest are high, but so are the impediments. No one would have predicted the skyrocket acceleration of the carve-out, and the carve-in may replicate such rapidity. We live in an era where changes in health care are unprecedented despite forces arrayed against them. The dismal record of the professional societies in stopping the previous changes attests to the fact there are scientific, professional, social, and economic forces that are mandat-

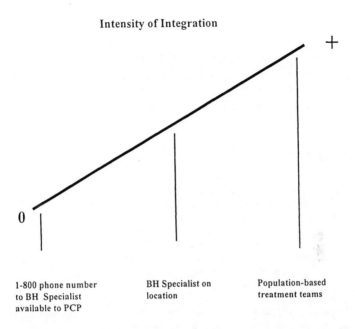

FIG. 7.2. Scale of intensity (degree) of integration of behavioral health with primary care. The 1-800 phone number to a behavioral health specialist is the simplest level, the behavioral health specialist on location is the midpoint, and population- and disease-based teams with obliteration of traditional departments represent the highest level. Most programs (clinical dependency, depression, lifestyle, etc.) fall below the midpoint of integration.

ing change. One thing is for certain: the changes over the next decade will be as profound as those of the preceding decade and will be different from anything we have ever seen.

SUMMARY

For a number of reasons, not only did psychology miss the first wave in the industrialization of behavioral health care, but also in its initial denial and later fury, its professional society, the APA, even rendered itself irrelevant to the profound decisions that were being made in U.S. health care during the past decade. The threshold of the second wave in the industrialization of behavioral health care has arrived, with changes that will be even greater than those of the first wave. There is once again opportunity and challenge for practitioners who are astute, bold, and visionary.

The new era favoring the practitioner stems from the mistakes the MCOs have made, on the one hand, and the new purchasing arrangements that enable the practitioner to bypass the MCOs and contract directly on the other. IDSs are being established throughout the nation and are successfully competing with the managed care companies. A second form of integration, that of behavioral health with primary care, is in its infancy, but promises to profoundly change not only health care, but psychology as well. The far-sighted practitioners are beginning now to become equity participants in the health care delivery system of the next decade. In the immediate future opportunities abound, but the window will not remain open indefinitely. The future lies with those psychologists who fill the new roles and who redefine behavioral health practice.

REFERENCES

Ackley, D. C. (1997). *Breaking free of managed care.* New York: Guilford.

Cummings, N. A. (1986). The dismantling of our health system: Strategies for the survival of psychological practice. *American Psychologist, 41,* 426–431.

Cummings, N. A. (1988). Emergence of the mental health complex: Adaptive and maladaptive responses. *Professional Psychology: Research and Practice, 19*(3), 308–315.

Cummings, N. A. (1995). Behavioral health after managed care: The next golden opportunity for professional psychology. *Register Report, 20*(3), 1, 30–32.

Cummings, N. A. (1996). The search for capital: Positioning for growth, joint venturing, acquisition, and public offering. In N. A. Cummings, M. S. Pallak, & J. L. Cummings (Eds.), *Surviving the demise of solo practice: Mental health practitioners prospering in the era of managed care* (pp. 205–217). Madison, CT: Psychosocial Press.

Cummings, N. A. (1997a). Behavioral health in primary care: Dollars and sense. In N. A. Cummings, J. L. Cummings, & J. N. Johnson, *Behavioral health in primary care: A guide for clinical integration* (pp. 3–22). Madison, CT: Psychosocial Press.

Cummings, N. A. (1997b, July/August). Practitioner-driven IDS groups continue as best hope for the future. *National Psychologist,* 10–11.

Cummings, N. A., Cummings, J. L., & Johnson, J. N. (1997). *Behavioral health in primary care: A guide for clinical integration.* Madison, CT: Psychosocial Press.

Cummings, N. A., & Fernandez, L. (1985, March). Exciting new opportunities for psychologists in the market place. *Independent Practitioner, 5,* 38–42.

Cummings, N. A., Pallak, M. S., & Cummings, J. L. (1996). *Surviving the demise of solo of solo practice: Mental health practitioners prospering in the era of managed care.* Madison, CT: Psychosocial Press.

Cummings, N., & Sayama, M. (1995). *Focused psychotherapy: A casebook of brief, intermittent psychotherapy throughout the life cycle.* Madison, CT: Psychosocial Press.

Drotos, J. C. (1997). Upheavals in the land of the giants. *Behavioral Health Management, 17*(8), 39–40.

Edley, R. S. (1996). The practitioner as owner. In N. A. Cummings, M. S. Pallak, & J. L. Cummings (eds.), *Surviving the demise of solo practice: Mental health practitioners prospering in the era of managed care* (pp. 175–190). Madison, CT: Psychosocial Press.

Jeffrey, N. A. (1998, January 5). A new balancing act for psychotherapy. *Wall Street Journal,* pp. B6, B7.

Joseph, S. (1997). *Symptom focused psychiatric drug therapy for managed care.* New York: Haworth.

Managed care defenders map an offensive against legislative mandates. (1998, January 16), *Wall Street Journal,* p. 1.

Newsline: Practitioners report decrease in earnings, (1997, March), *APA Monitor, 28*(3), p. 6.

Oss, M. E. (1997, November/December). Business strategy: Foundation for the future. *Behavioral Healthcare Management,* 17(8), 4.

Peaks and valleys. (December 1997), *Practice Strategies,* 3(12), 1 & 12.

Pullham, S., & Winslow, R. (1997, October 9). HMO bleeding is unsettling Wall Street. *Wall Street Journal,* pp. C1, C2.

Ross, C., Covall, M., Graham, M., & Coakley, T. (1998, January 15). Experts predict consolidation fall-out, provider-sponsored networks, shrinking behavioral health dollars in 1998. *Managed Behavioral Health News,* pp. 1–4.

Ross, E. C. (1997, December 7). Plans present mixed bag of results for providers, subscribers. *Tallahassee Democrat,* pp. F1, F4.

Sherer, R. A. (1997). HMO cost comparison study. *Mental Health Economics,* 1(1), 1–2.

Sherrid, P. (1997). Mismanaged care? Wall Street takes the scalpel to HMO companies. *U. S. News & World Report,* November 24, 57–62.

Stoil, M. J. (1997, November/December). Parity: Case closed? *Behavioral Health Management,* 17(8), 6–7.

Valdmanis, T. (1998, January 2). Mega-mergers likely to contain momentum. *USA Today,* B1, B6.

Weinstein, M., & Edley, R. S. (1997, February). Whither the solo and the group practice? *Behavioral Healthcare Tomorrow,* 1(6), 39–43.

Author Index

163

Gurman, A. S., 27, 55, 135

H

Hammeke, T. A., 25
Harwood, T. M., 29
Henault, K., 58
Hendren, J., 12
Hennessey, S., 92
Hermann, B., 58
Hersch, L., 11, 17
Hidalgo, J., 90
Hoag, M. J., 69
Holstein, L., 44, 118
Hornberger, J., 76
Howard, K. I., 48, 67, 68
Hoyt, M. F., 8, 11, 41, 43, 45, 48, 54,
    113, 118, 136
Humphreys, K., 114
Hunter, R., 50
Hurt, S. W., 28

I

Imber, S. D., 32

J

Jeffrey, N. A., 154
Johnson, J. N., 147, 157, 158
Johnson, P., 110
Joseph, S., 141
Joyce, A. S., 69

K

Kachele, H., 68
Kaplan, R. M., 33
Karno, M., 137
Karon, B., 7
Karp, J. F., 122
Kashner, T., 90
Katon, W., 90, 92, 98, 99, 105
Kelleher, K., 33
Kent, A., 8, 10
Kin, E. J., 137
Kisch, J., 45
Klein, A., 36
Kleinke, C., 50

Klerman, G. L., 32, 67
Klump, K., 24
Knapp, S., 44
Kobos, J. C., 46, 50
Kohout, J., 118, 119, 126, 127, 128,
    130, 136
Kohrman, C. H., 44
Kopta, S. M., 68
Koss, M. P., 43, 123
Krause, M. S., 67
Kroenke, K., 90

L

Lambart, M., 45, 46
Lambert, M. J., 43, 68, 125
Lambert, M. L., 28
Langbehn, D. R., 36
Larson, D., 90
Lazar, S.G., 76
Leber, W. R., 32
Levenson, H., 113, 116, 117, 122, 123,
    124, 125, 134, 137
Levin, B. L., 48
Lin, E., 90, 92, 98, 99, 105
Locke, B., 89
Lowry, J. L., 68
Ludman, E., 92, 98, 99, 105
Lueger, R. J., 68
Lunnen, K. M., 125

M

MacDonald, R., 3
Machado, P. P., 31
MacKenzie, K. R., 9, 66, 67, 70, 71, 72
Mahoney, M. T., 48
Manderscheid, R., 89
Mangelsdorf, A., 90
Martin, S., 3
Matier-Sharma, K., 26
McGuire, P., 3
McGuire, T., 46
McMahon, T. C., 44
McRoberts, C., 69
Mckay, M., 74
Meredith, K., 31
Mergenthaler, E., 68
Merry, W., 31
Mesh, S., 3

Subject Index

A

Achenbach Child Behavior Checklist, 25
Aetna Life and Casualty, 149
American Managed Behavioral Health care Association (AMBHA), 146–147, 154
American Psych Systems, 149
American Psychological Association, 3–4
Assessment and Testing and, 23–39
  promotion of, 24–25
  roles of, 25–37
    enhancing treatment quality and outcome, 28–32
    in evaluation of treatment outcomes, 35–36
    in primary care settings, 32–35
    reduction in treatment length, 27–28
    traditional, 25–27
Attention Deficit Hyperactivity Disorder (ADHD), 25–26
Attitudes Regarding Managed Care, 75–77, 124–125

B

Beck Scales for Depression and Anxiety, 28, 32–33, 36
Brief Symptom Index, 32
Bureau of Veterans Affairs, 115

C

Center for Mental Health Services (CMHS), 121
Challenges of, an Overview, 7–10, 75–81
  administrative, 9–10
  clinical, 8–9
  professional, 10
Cognitive Behavior Therapy (CBT), 73
Columbia/HCA, 143, 149, 151
Conference of Graduate Education and Training in Psychology, 116
Conners Ratings Scales, 25

D

Department of Justice, 143
Department of Veterans Affairs, 133
Diagnostic and Statistical Manual of Mental Disorders (DSM–IV), 32, 36

F

Family Enterprises, 149
FHC Options, 149
First Mental Health, 149
Foster Higgins, 145
Foundation Health PsychCare, 149
FPM Behavioral Health, 149
Future of, an Overview, 12–17

For Product Safety Concerns and Information please contact our EU
representative GPSR@taylorandfrancis.com Taylor & Francis Verlag GmbH,
Kaufingerstraße 24, 80331 München, Germany

Printed and bound by CPI Group (UK) Ltd, Croydon, CR0 4YY

10/06/2025

01898421-0001